Operation Health

Operation Health

Surgical Care in the Developing World

Edited by
ADAM L. KUSHNER, MD, MPH, FACS

Johns Hopkins University Press
Baltimore

© 2015 Johns Hopkins University Press
All rights reserved. Published 2015
Printed in the United States of America on acid-free paper
2 4 6 8 9 7 5 3 1

Johns Hopkins University Press
2715 North Charles Street
Baltimore, Maryland 21218-4363
www.press.jhu.edu

Library of Congress Cataloging-in-Publication Data

Operation health : surgical care in the developing world /
edited by Adam L. Kushner.
p. ; cm.
Includes bibliographical references and index.
ISBN 978-1-4214-1669-4 (paperback : alk. paper)—ISBN 1-4214-1669-7
(paperback : alk. paper)—ISBN 978-1-4214-1670-0 (electronic)—
ISBN 1-4214-1670-0 (electronic)
I. Kushner, Adam L., 1965– , editor.
[DNLM: 1. Developing Countries—Case Reports. 2. Surgical Procedures,
Operative—Case Reports. 3. General Surgery—education—Case Reports.
4. Health Services Accessibility—Case Reports. 5. Quality of
Health Care—Case Reports. WA 395]
RD31.5
617.09172′4—dc23
2014029351

A catalog record for this book is available from the British Library.

Special discounts are available for bulk purchases of this book. For more information,
please contact Special Sales at 410-516-6936 or specialsales@press.jhu.edu.

Johns Hopkins University Press uses environmentally friendly book materials,
including recycled text paper that is composed of at least 30 percent
post-consumer waste, whenever possible.

CONTENTS

Tigistu Adamu Ashengo, MD, MPH
Associate Medical Director
Jhpiego
Baltimore, MD, USA

Olusegun I. Alatise, MD
Department of Surgery
Division of Gastrointestinal/Surgical
   Oncology
Obafemi Awolowo University/Teaching
   Hospitals Complex
Ile-Ife, Osun, Nigeria

Jean Anderson, MD
Department of Gynecology
   and Obstetrics
Johns Hopkins Hospital
Baltimore, MD, USA

Ashok K. Banskota, MD
Hospital and Rehabilitation
   Centre for Disabled Children
Kavre, Janagal, Nepal

Bibek Banskota, MD
Hospital and Rehabilitation Centre for
   Disabled Children
Kavre, Janagal, Nepal

Gabriel Boakye, MB, ChB
Department of Anesthesia
Komfo Anokye Teaching Hospital
Kumasi, Ghana

Respicious Boniface, MD, MMED, MSC
Muhimbili Orthopaedic Institute
Muhimbili University of Health and
   Allied Sciences
Injury Control Centre Tanzania
Dar es Salaam, Tanzania

Amber Caldwell, BA
Department of Orthopaedic
   Surgery, University of California, San
   Francisco (UCSF), CA, USA
Institute for Global Orthopaedics and
   Traumatology, San Francisco, CA, USA
Department of Orthopaedic Surgery,
   San Francisco General Hospital
   (SFGH), San Francisco, CA, USA
UCSF SFGH Orthopaedic Trauma
   Institute, San Francisco, CA, USA

Anthony Charles, MD, MPH, FACS
Associate Professor of Surgery, University
   of North Carolina School of Medicine,
   Chapel Hill, NC, USA
Adjunct Associate Professor of
   Public Health, Gillings School of
   Global Public Health, University
   of North Carolina at Chapel Hill,
   Chapel Hill, NC, USA

Program Director, UNC-Malawi Surgical
  Initiative, University of North Carolina
  at Chapel Hill, Chapel Hill, NC, USA

Marc Dakermandji, MD
Centre for Global Surgery
McGill University Health Centre
Montreal, Quebec, Canada

Dan L. Deckelbaum, MD, MPH
Co-director
Centre for Global Surgery
McGill University Health Centre
Montreal, Quebec, Canada

Iain Elliott, MD
Department of Orthopaedic Surgery,
  University of California, San Francisco
  (UCSF), CA, USA
Institute for Global Orthopaedics
  and Traumatology, San Francisco,
  CA, USA
Department of Orthopaedic Surgery, San
  Francisco General Hospital (SFGH),
  San Francisco, CA, USA
UCSF SFGH Orthopaedic Trauma
  Institute, San Francisco, CA, USA

Heather L. Gill, MD, MPH
Centre for Global Surgery
McGill University Health Centre
Montreal, Quebec, Canada

Richard A. Gosselin, MD, MPH
Department of Orthopaedic Surgery,
  University of California, San Francisco
  (UCSF), CA, USA
Institute for Global Orthopaedics and
  Traumatology, San Francisco, CA, USA
Department of Orthopaedic Surgery, San
  Francisco General Hospital (SFGH),
  San Francisco, CA, USA
UCSF SFGH Orthopaedic Trauma
  Institute, San Francisco, CA, USA

Reinou S. Groen, MD, MIH, PhD
Department of Gynecology
  and Obstetrics
Johns Hopkins Hospital
Baltimore, MD, USA

Mark Harris, MD
Associate Professor
Department of Anesthesiology
University of Utah Hospital
Salt Lake City, UT, USA

T. Peter Kingham, MD
Assistant Professor, Division of
  Hepatopancreatobiliary Surgery,
  Memorial Sloan-Kettering Cancer
  Center, New York, NY, USA
President, Surgeons OverSeas, New York,
  NY, USA

Adam L. Kushner, MD, MPH, FACS
Surgeons OverSeas, New York, NY, USA
Department of Surgery, Columbia
  University, New York, NY, USA
Department of International Health,
  Johns Hopkins Bloomberg School of
  Public Health, Baltimore, MD, USA

Benedict C. Nwomeh, MD, MPH
Professor of Surgery and Pediatrics,
  Associate Academic Program Director
  for Foundational Sciences, Ohio State
  University College of Medicine,
  Columbus, OH, USA
Program Director for Pediatric Surgery,
  Medical Director, International Visiting
  Scholars Program, Nationwide
  Children's Hospital, Columbus,
  OH, USA

Juliet S. Okoroh, MD, MPH
Resident in General Surgery
University of California
San Francisco, CA, USA

Lauren Owens, MD, MPH
Department of Gynecology
   and Obstetrics
Johns Hopkins Hospital
Baltimore, MD, USA

Kushal R. Patel, MD
Department of Orthopaedic Surgery,
   University of California, San Francisco
   (UCSF), San Francisco, CA, USA
Institute for Global Orthopaedics and
   Traumatology, San Francisco, CA, USA
Department of Orthopaedic Surgery, San
   Francisco General Hospital (SFGH),
   San Francisco, CA, USA
UCSF SFGH Orthopaedic Trauma
   Institute, San Francisco, CA, USA

Raymond R. Price, MD
Director of Graduate Surgical Education,
   Intermountain Surgical Specialists,
   Intermountain Healthcare, Salt Lake
   City, UT, USA
Associate Director, Center for Global
   Surgery, University of Utah, Salt Lake
   City, UT, USA
Adjunct Associate Professor, Department
   of Surgery, University of Utah, Salt
   Lake City, UT, USA
Adjunct Associate Professor, Department
   of Family and Preventive Medicine,
   Division of Public Health, University of
   Utah, Salt Lake City, UT, USA

Tarun Rajbhandary, MD
Hospital and Rehabilitation Centre for
   Disabled Children
Kavre, Janagal, Nepal

Tarek Razek, MD
Co-director
Centre for Global Surgery
McGill University Health Centre
Montreal, Quebec, Canada

Orgoi Sergelen, MD, PhD
Chief of Surgery
Department of Surgery
Health Sciences University of Mongolia
Ulaanbaatar, Mongolia

Om P. Shrestha, MD
Hospital and Rehabilitation Centre for
   Disabled Children
Kavre, Janagal, Nepal

David A. Spiegel, MD
Division of Orthopaedic Surgery,
   Children's Hospital of Philadelphia,
   Philadelphia, PA, USA
Associate Professor of Orthopaedic
   Surgery, University of Pennsylvania
   School of Medicine, Philadelphia, PA,
   USA

Carlos Varela, MD
Chief of Surgery
Department of Surgery
Kamuzu Central Hospital
Lilongwe, Malawi

Evan G. Wong, MD, MPH
Centre for Global Surgery, McGill
   University Health Centre, Montreal,
   Quebec, Canada
Surgeons OverSeas, New York, NY,
   USA

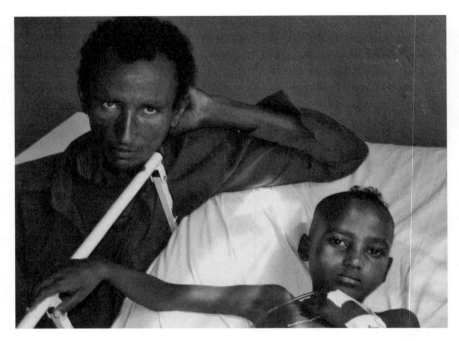

Figure P.1. Recovering from an operation, Ethiopia.
Photo courtesy Adam L. Kushner

Imagine a child falling from a tree and being disabled for life; a young man dying from appendicitis or a strangulated hernia; a woman dying in childbirth or, after delivering a dead baby, being left with the continuous leakage of urine or stool from an obstetric fistula. These conditions are so rare in high-income countries (HICs) that they are typically not seen outside of textbooks. In low- and middle-income countries (LMICs), these conditions are unfortunately everyday occurrences and not only treatable but preventable.

With a simple cast, a child's broken bone can heal properly; with an appendectomy or hernia repair, a wage earner can again be a productive member of society; with a cesarean section, a woman and her child can survive a difficult pregnancy or avoid an obstetric fistula.

In HICs, surgical care is so accessible and relied upon that there is rarely a second thought about seeking attention for a broken bone, deep cut, burn, congenital deformity, difficult pregnancy, or cancerous growth. But with all the benefits that surgery can provide for patients and populations, few international health researchers focus on surgical care. Why? When an estimated two billion people around the world lack access to an operating room, why is it that surgery is not considered to be an integral part of health systems? Where is the support for surgical care from donors and aid agencies? Where are the governments, academics, civil society organizations, and businesses that can help prevent millions of deaths and hundreds of millions of permanent disabilities? There is a saying among surgeons that "a chance to cut is a chance to cure," but surgical care is much more than mere cutting. Within the global surgery community, surgical care is defined as wound care—suturing, incision, excision, or otherwise manipulating tissue—in a safe and painless way. From the perspective of an individual patient or a population, surgery is a chance to prevent, diagnose, treat, and palliate disease.

This book highlights various topics relating to global surgery, and presents case studies and best practices from surgical and public health experts from around the world. These specialists and their international colleagues seek to distill their experiences and identify what worked, what did not, and why.

Each chapter begins with a short personal vignette by the volume editor, a personal recollection of a case or conversation to help frame the issue. Specific case studies follow a basic public health approach to problem solving: define a problem, measure its magnitude, identify the key determinants, propose interventions, set priorities, describe interventions and evaluations, and make plans for the future. The aim of this book is to educate and inspire. The cases are real, and countless lives have been saved by surgical care. As word spreads that surgery can prevent, diagnose, treat, and palliate, it is hoped that policymakers and donors will understand the needs, benefits, and urgency of improving access to surgical care globally.

REFERENCES

Funk LM, Weiser TG, Berry WR, et al. Global operating theatre distribution and pulse oximetry supply: an estimation from reported data. *Lancet.* 2010; 376(9746): 1055–61.

Kushner AL, Kingham TP, Nwomeh BC. Medicine and surgery: the yin and yang of health systems. *Lancet.* 2012; 379(9825): 1488.

This book is the result of the experiences and dedication of many people. I wish to thank all the chapter contributors for their effort, support, and desire to help patients needing surgical care around the world. They are true experts in the field of global surgery, and I am proud to call them my friends.

I also want to thank all the patients in whose care I was able to participate, and to acknowledge the millions of patients around the world who die or remain disabled because of a lack of surgical care. It is my hope that this work will in a small way help improve access to care.

Pursuing an atypical surgical career path has required a great deal of support and encouragement from many people. Numerous mentors were essential during my surgical training. Morris D. Kerstein, MD, former chairman of surgery at Hahnemann University in Philadelphia, was an early and strong supporter of my plans to work globally. Joel J. Roslyn, MD, former chairman of surgery at Allegheny University of the Health Sciences in Philadelphia, believed in me and allowed me to pursue a master of public health. As an MPH student at the Johns Hopkins Bloomberg School of Public Health in Baltimore, I met Gilbert M. Burnham, MD, PhD, professor of international health. He taught me about humanitarian assistance and gave me the sage advice to, when planning to operate on patients in a low-resource setting, "Make sure they have a blood pressure before you begin." He also helped initiate the course "Surgical Care Needs in Low- and Middle-Income Countries," out of which this book developed.

Others I wish to thank include Mark A. Hardy, MD, Auchincloss Professor of Surgery at the Columbia University College of Physicians and Surgeons in New York, who provided tireless support and friendship and who has a keen interest in expanding surgical care around the world. Arturo P. Muyco, MD, former chief of surgery at Kamuzu Central Hospital in Lilongwe, Malawi, taught me most of what I know about global surgery, and Thaim B. Kamara, MD, chief of surgery at Connaught Hospital in Freetown, Sierra Leone, taught me much of the rest. I thank them both for their dedication and clinical excellence, amazing work in difficult environments, mentorship, and friendship.

Lastly, I wish to thank my parents, Zina and Daniel B. Kushner, MD, for their love and support as well as my wife, global surgery partner, and best friend, Reinou S. Groen, MD, MIH, PhD, for her love, support, and encouragement.

Operation Health

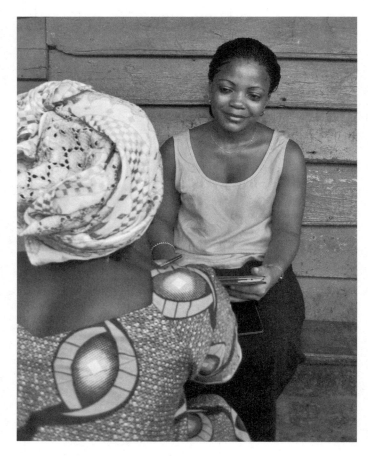

Figure 1.1. Collecting surgical data, Sierra Leone.
Photo courtesy Reinou S. Groen

CHAPTER ONE

Quantifying the Need for Surgical Care

A Case Study from Sierra Leone

REINOU S. GROEN, MD, MIH, PHD

Without the relatively simple operation, the father of three and main breadwinner of the family would certainly have died. He presented to the hospital like so many other patients in low- and middle-income countries (LMICs), with nearly dead intestines stuck in a defect in his abdominal wall—a condition known as a strangulated hernia. In high-income countries, such conditions are uncommon and rarely fatal; hernias are usually repaired early to prevent strangulation. In LMICs, millions of hernias remain unrepaired, with strangulation and death being all too common.

That patient survived. His case was followed by that of another young man, who presented with signs of a ruptured appendix. In the operating room, more than a gallon of pus was drained. The rupture had occurred five days previously; luckily, he had been strong enough to survive the long journey to the hospital. He too would survive.

Traditional public health teaching does not routinely include surgical care, but untreated hernias and appendicitis are only two examples of surgically treatable conditions that have received little attention from the global health community. Questions emerged as a result of caring for a multitude of patients with these conditions. Could such situations have been prevented? If these were the strong patients who survived, how many patients died before reaching the hospital? What was the surgical need of the population? What was the magnitude of the problem?

To begin to truly address the presumed massive surgical need throughout the world, a public health approach was needed. The problem, which in LMICs could be defined only by extrapolating data from hospital records, was two billion people without access to surgical care, millions dying, and hundreds of millions permanently disabled from treatable conditions. But the specifics of the problem at the community level were completely unknown. A population-based household survey of surgical need was required to determine a "denominator," or the number of people in the population who suffer with or die from a surgically treatable condition.

This need for a baseline led to the development of a collaborative effort by academic institutions, ministries of health, and civil society organizations to create a tool—a survey—to estimate the prevalence of surgical care needs before addressing the problem.

Surgical care is not always acknowledged as a requirement in global health, and the reasons why are varied. First, many public health and global health efforts were initially based on the prevention or eradication of communicable or infectious diseases, with surgical care viewed as strictly a curative process. Second, until recently, few surgeons were involved in public health and global health efforts owing to a lack of interest, time, or exposure to public health techniques. Third, surgical care was considered too expensive of an investment that necessitated a large commitment requiring too many resources. Last, only limited epidemiological data on the surgical needs of populations in LMICs were available to document the problem.

In an effort to strengthen surgical care in LMICs, Surgeons OverSeas (SOS), a nongovernmental organization, was founded in 2007. The SOS mission is to save lives in developing countries by improving surgical care. As part of its mandate, SOS has provided technical and financial support to local surgeons, hospitals, and ministries of health in LMICs to assist in building long-term surgical capacity. SOS programs concentrate on life-saving and disability-preventing procedures that can be undertaken and taught in resource-limited environments.

Surgeons OverSeas has also been active in research and advocacy at the local government and international levels. Research has helped to document and understand available resources for providing surgical care. A surgical capacity survey and index, the PIPES tool—personnel, infrastructure, procedures, equipment, and supplies—which assesses surgical health facilities, was developed to easily document baseline conditions and to assist in developing intervention strategies. All collected data are shared with local surgeons and ministries of health and then published in peer-reviewed journals.

To broaden knowledge of the need for surgical care, a research strategy to estimate the incidence and prevalence of surgically treatable conditions was envisioned. Because only scattered data collected by inconsistent methodologies existed, a need was identified for a global replicable countrywide assessment tool. The tool had to be useful to investigate the epidemiology of surgical needs in countries where surgical care is limited and clinical databases are sparse or nonexistent. Therefore the Surgeons OverSeas Assessment of Surgical Need (SO-SAS), a population-based community survey, was developed. Figure 1.2 illustrates the overall survey design process.

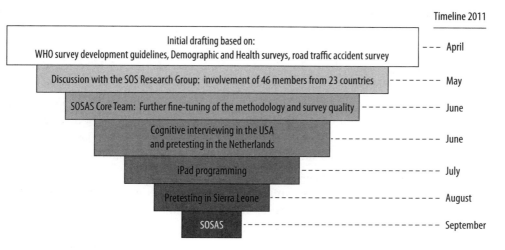

Figure 1.2. Surgeons OverSeas Assessment of Surgical Need, or SOSAS, survey tool development and timeline.

In creating SOSAS, an initial draft questionnaire was developed on the basis of World Health Organization guidelines, the Demographic and Health Surveys (DHSs), and a survey of road traffic incidents. The included conditions had to be easily recognizable by laypersons, have a significant incidence and prevalence, and have a potential for treatment with available local resources. Questions were developed to address surgical needs and were structured to fit into broader categories, such as wounds, masses, burns, and congenital and acquired deformities, as well as a group of symptoms such as recurrent discharge from an arm or leg to indicate a chronic bone infection (osteomyelitis), rectal bleeding for possible colorectal cancer, and constant leaking of urine or feces as a proxy for an obstetric fistula.

A research group from SOS consisting of 46 surgeons, public health experts, nurses, medical students, and residents from academic and rural medical centers in 23 countries commented on the draft survey. Discussions also led to a decision to use iPads to collect the data. The arguments against using high-tech devices included the initial investment costs, need for programming, possible breakage or theft, and training on device usage. The arguments for using iPads proved to be overwhelming and included better standardization of the methodology, facilitation of collecting and recording of data, easier statistical analysis and evaluations, and better data control and conditional formatting. The use of iPads even had the potential to reduce study costs, as less printing and no subsequent data entry would be required. Additionally, data analysis would be available throughout the data collection process, which would give instant feedback to the interviewers.

Collaboration with the University of Virginia Center for Survey Research led to the establishment of a survey methodology. Cognitive interviewing and pretesting occurred prior to a pilot study and subsequent implementation in Sierra Leone. Comments from the ethical review board of the Royal Tropical Institute in the Netherlands and personnel at Statistics Sierra Leone (SSL) and the College of Medicine and Allied Health Sciences in Sierra Leone helped to fine-tune the survey tool and methodology.

Sierra Leone was chosen as an initial site for the study because SOS had a long-standing relationship with the local surgical community and the Ministry of Health and Sanitation. A small West African country with a population of six million, in 2011 Sierra Leone ranked 180th of the 187 nations on the United Nations Human Development Index, with a gross national income of $340 per person per year and over 70% of the population living in poverty. The major health indicators for Sierra Leone revealed that life expectancy at birth was 48 years, an estimated 174 per 1,000 children died before their fifth birthday, and maternal mortality rates were among the highest in the world.

For the execution of the survey, several priorities were set. First, the research would cover a representative sample of the country and would produce high-quality data usable by the Sierra Leone Ministry of Health and Sanitation and for publication in peer-reviewed journals.

To be representative or to have external validity, a sample needs to reflect all groups within a population, including representative age, sex, and social and economic distributions. In the case of Sierra Leone, 14 different tribes are present, and rural and urban areas are quite different; therefore these differences were taken into account by stratification of the sample for all the districts and for rural versus urban areas when randomly assigning the clusters. Each cluster had approximately 80–120 households, requiring a second step of randomization to allow the assessment of more clusters for greater diversity in the sample; however, not all 80–120 households in each cluster had to be interviewed. This two-stage cluster-based sampling technique is well known and, combined with cluster selection with a chance proportional to population size, makes the overall results a weighted sample. Clusters with a greater numbers of households are more likely to be chosen to begin with, but because only 25 households were going to be assessed, in the larger clusters, each individual household had a lower chance of being selected.

Because no population-based data on surgically treatable conditions in LMICs were previously available, the sample size calculation was based on a 7.3% prevalence of surgical need identified by the pilot test of 100 individuals conducted in Sierra Leone in August 2011. For the full country survey, a sample size of 3,745 responses was determined to be necessary.

For the SOSAS survey in Sierra Leone, nurses, medical and nursing students, and employees from SSL who had previously participated in multiple DHSs were recruited as survey interviewers and received five days of training on the survey tool, use of the iPads, interview techniques, and respondent selection. The training included translational aspects, multiple mock interviews, and one field exercise where all the survey interviewers interviewed at least one household. The field supervisors were included in the training and met with the principal investigator each day to discuss progress and make logistical preparations to execute the survey.

Survey interviewers were divided into five teams for data collection in the districts on the basis of their language skills, and each team had at least one member from SSL with previous experience in locating enumerating areas (EAs), which were the smallest census designations randomly selected as clusters for the survey. Each team received a vehicle, driver, first aid kit, iPads and chargers, and per diem allotments for food and lodging.

Once in the field, after identification of the randomly preselected EA, teams contacted the chief of the village or section and sought permission to conduct the study. To select households within each cluster, a structure count—in which each structure was numbered—was first performed and then an initial house was randomly selected. Every fifth structure was subsequently chosen until a total of 25 households were interviewed. If more than one household lived in a structure, a single household was randomly chosen from that structure after listing the household leaders. Household members were defined as those who ate from the same pot and slept in the same structure the night before the interview, as is the definition for the DHS in Sierra Leone.

A supervisor with each team regularly checked the completed surveys for inconsistencies as well as completeness. The teams completed data collection in 15 days.

Seventy-four of the randomly selected clusters were located and confirmed by GPS coordinates. One cluster could not be located because of outdated information on the EA map and was replaced with a village in the same chiefdom. Of the 1,875 total targeted households, data were obtained for 1,843 households. Data from 25 households surveyed on the first interview day, which was also part of the training workshop, were not included. In addition, two households refused to give consent for the survey, and five households contained too much missing information and were therefore not included in the analysis.

The survey teams attempted to interview two members of each household. The total expected number of interviews was determined to be 3,686. In 41 cases (1.1%), however, only one household member was interviewed, and for 21 respondents, data were missing on essential questions for the outcome of this research. Thus the total number of responses was 3,624. Of note, 149 (4.1%) of selected household members were replaced, as the persons initially identified were not available for interview even after revisiting the structure on multiple occasions. A full selection of data was ultimately collected and analyzed from 1,843 households and 3,645 respondents, giving a response rate of 98.3%. The majority of household interviews were completed on the initial visit ($n = 1,696$). Two visits were required for 132 households, and 15 households required three visits before the interviews could be completed.

Of the 3,645 respondents, 1,352 (37%) indicated that they had a wound, burn, mass, growth, deformity, or other surgical condition at the time of the interview, and 896 (25%) indicated that they were in need of surgical care. Five hundred and seventy-five households reported having at least one deceased household member in the previous year, for a total of 709 deaths. Of these households, 471 reported one death in the last year, 78 reported two, 22 reported three, and four reported four deaths in the last year. Based on the symptoms reported in the week prior to death, a total of 237 (33.4%) deaths possibly resulted from surgical conditions. These symptoms were categorized as abdominal distention and pain (98), death during childbirth (42), injury (41), mass (21), acquired deformity (18), non-injury-related wound (10), and congenital deformity (7). Of the 237 deaths with a surgical condition as defined in the categories, 58 indicated that there was "no need" for a surgical intervention, resulting in a total of 179 deaths (25.2%; confidence interval 22.5%–27.9%) out of 709 that may have benefited from surgical care before death.

The data clearly show a high prevalence of untreated surgical conditions in Sierra Leone. The final analysis demonstrated that 25% of respondents had a condition that likely required at minimum a surgical consultation. The survey also showed that 25% of deaths identified in the previous year could possibly have been prevented with adequate access to surgical services. If one were to extrapolate the findings to the entire population of Sierra Leone, an estimated 1.5 million individuals would have benefited from a surgical consultation at the time of the study.

The Surgeons OverSeas Assessment of Surgical Need was also used for a national assessment of surgical need in Rwanda, a country with greater financial support and considered to be more advanced on the development scale than Sierra Leone. In Rwanda, 6.4% (95%; confidence interval, 5.6%–7.3%) of the population was found to need a surgical evaluation. Using the lower confidence interval for surgical need in Rwanda and a population estimate of one billion people in sub-Saharan Africa, it can be extrapolated that 56 million people are currently in need of surgical evaluation and will most likely need an intervention.

The major limitations of the SOSAS studies were that the findings relied solely on verbal interviews of self-reported conditions and were not confirmed by physical examinations or chart reviews. The respondents' perception of a surgical condition might not be correct. A mass caused by Burkitt's lymphoma, for example, which is endemic in certain countries, would need chemotherapy rather than a surgical procedure. Despite this reservation, the interviewers, when debriefed, found that a majority of interviewees were quite knowledgeable about what constitutes a surgical condition. This finding was consistent with qualitative research from focus-group discussions performed in Sierra Leone at the same time.

Some critics have questioned the use of such surveys and the cost of implementation in light of scarce resources in LMICs. But the SOSAS study was relatively inexpensive—only $35,000 per country—and provided high-quality and important data essential to distributing scarce health-care resources and planning interventions.

When planning similar studies in the future, it is highly recommended that a pilot test first be completed. This short test will help obtain insight into how to use the questionnaire and which questions may not be appropriate; identify community and national contacts; plan day-to-day logistics; ascertain the most effective execution plan; and assist with staff selection before undertaking the full country study. Experience from the SOSAS study confirmed the advice of Seymour Sudman and Norman M. Bradburn that "If you do not have the resources to pilot test your questionnaire, don't do the study."

In looking toward the future and the most effective and practical methods of delivering surgical health care in LMICs, each country must define its own burden of surgical disease profile. When results of similar studies become available, it may be possible to correlate them with the United Nations Human Development Index or gross national income. Doing so may not only be highly informative, but it may also permit the development of interventions suitable for individual countries. Identification of health-care system determinants (e.g., governmental systems vs. private systems) will also provide critical insights for the most effective and practical way to provide surgical care for populations in need.

Note: The SOSAS survey is available online at www.surgeonsoverseas.org/resources.html.

REFERENCES

Courtright P, Haile D, Kohls E. The epidemiology of burns in rural Ethiopia. *J Epidemiol Com Health.* 1993; 47(1): 19–22.

Groen RS, Sriram VM, Kamara TB, Kushner AL, Blok L. Individual and community perceptions of surgical care in Sierra Leone. *Trop Med Int Health.* 2014; 19(1): 107–16.

Guerrero A, Amegashie J, Obiri-Yeboah M, Appiah N, Zakariah A. Paediatric road traffic injuries in urban Ghana: a population-based study. *Inj Prev.* 2011; 17(5): 309–12.

Kelsey JL. *Methods in Observational Epidemiology.* 2nd ed. New York: Oxford University Press; 1996: 337.

Mock CN, Abantanga F, Cummings P, Koepsell PD. Incidence and outcome of injury in Ghana: a community based survey. *Bull World Health Organ.* 1999; 77(12): 955–64.

Nordberg E. Incidence and estimated need of caesarean section, inguinal hernia repair, and operation for strangulated hernia in rural Africa. *Br Med J (Clin Res Ed).* 1984; 289(6437): 92–93.

———. Injuries as a public health problem in sub-Saharan Africa: epidemiology and prospects for control. *East Afr Med J.* 2000; 77: S1-43.

UN Development Programme. International human development indicators: Sierra Leone. http://hdr.undp.org/sites/default/files/Country-Profiles/SLE.pdf. Accessed June 26, 2014.

World Health Organization. Global Health Observatory, Sierra Leone, country data and statistics. http://www.who.int/gho/countries/sle/en/. Accessed June 20, 2014.

Zimmerman K, Mzige AA, Kibatala PL, Museru LM, Guerrero A. Road traffic injury incidence and crash characteristics in Dar es Salaam: a population based study. *Accid Anal Prev.* 2012; 45: 204–10.

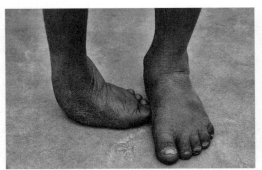

Figure 2.1. Neglected clubfoot, Malawi.
Photos courtesy Steve Mannion, Feet First 2012

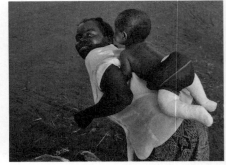

Figure 2.2. Malawian mother with child undergoing Ponseti clubfoot treatment.

JOHNS HOPKINS

Johns Hopkins University Press
2715 N. Charles Street
Baltimore MD 21218
www.press.jhu.edu

OPERATION HEALTH
Surgical Care in the Developing World

edited by Adam L. Kushner, MD, MPH, FACS

978-1-4214-1669-4 $25.95 paperback
978-1-4214-1670-0 $25.95 ebook

Publication Date: May 28, 2015

CHAPTER TWO

Children's Health

Clubfoot Repair in Nepal

DAVID A. SPIEGEL, MD, BIBEK BANSKOTA, MD,
OM P. SHRESTHA, MD, TARUN RAJBHANDARY, MD,
AND ASHOK K. BANSKOTA, MD

A pregnant woman in labor begins to bleed. Placenta previa—in which the placenta blocks the birth canal—is diagnosed. An emergent cesarean section saves the child and prevents the mother from bleeding to death. A few months later, the child projectile vomits repeatedly after eating. Pyloric stenosis—a muscular blockage of the small intestine—is diagnosed. An operation eliminates the blockage. A few years later, the child develops right-sided abdominal pain, fever, and nausea. Appendicitis is diagnosed, and an operation removes a gangrenous appendix. In many countries, millions of children have no access to such operations and die. Yet in high-income countries these three procedures are readily available and save lives. These three procedures saved my life; I was that child.

From stitches in the emergency room to cleft-lip repairs and resections of abdominal tumors, children frequently need access to surgical care. In fact, traumatic injuries are currently the leading cause of death for children aged 5 to 15, and millions more are permanently disabled because of a lack of surgical care.

To address the surgical needs of children around the world, a public health approach is needed. Clubfoot represents one success story of a devastating condition frequently seen in low- and middle-income countries (LMICs). Although clubfoot is treatable and correctable with a minimally invasive and relatively simple procedure, hundreds of thousands of untreated cases exist globally.

To help save and improve the lives of children around the world, we must identify what works from successful programs and expand those lessons to countless other conditions that affect people everywhere. This chapter describes a problem—children with clubfeet in Nepal—and a solution—a project to correct the deformity.

Congenital clubfoot (*talipes equinovarus*) is the most common congenital musculoskeletal deformity, occurring approximately once in every 1,000 live births. As such, tens of thousands of children live in LMICs with untreated clubfeet. While an untreated clubfoot makes it impossible to wear standard shoes and may also result in chronic pain, perhaps the most significant consequence is social stigma. Children with congenital clubfoot may be considered cursed, and in some societies it may be difficult if not impossible for a young lady with a clubfoot to get married. Given the incidence of clubfeet and the potential consequences, timely and effective treatment is ideal. Children diagnosed at the time of birth and can be referred for treatment by the Ponseti method if local resources are available.

The treatment of clubfoot has evolved over the past decades. From the 1970s through the 1990s, the most popular approach was serial casting followed by extensive soft-tissue release surgery. Long-term follow up of this approach often found stiff and painful feet with residual deformities. Additional surgical procedures were required in up to 50% of patients. In the 1950s, Ignacio Ponseti at the University of Iowa developed a minimally invasive approach. But it was not until the beginning of the 21st century that the Ponseti method gained popularity in the United States as a treatment method.

The Ponseti method has subsequently become a widely accepted technique throughout the world. It involves repeated casting, with approximately 90% of patients needing release of the heel cord tendon to complete the initial correction. Long leg casts are applied and changed at five- to seven-day intervals in young children. In older patients, some practitioners leave each cast on for two weeks. The last cast after the tendon release is kept on for three weeks, and then patients are transitioned to a brace program to maintain the correction. Brace programs involve wearing a foot brace for three months full time, and then at night up until the age of 5. Relapse of the clubfoot may happen in approximately 15% of patients and is treated by repeating the method. In children older than 2 to 3 years of age, relapse may be due to overactivity of the tibialis anterior muscle and is treated by repeating the Ponseti method and then adding a tendon transfer. Ultimately, this method is effective in greater than 90% of patients presenting in infancy.

For the Ponseti method to be effective in a population, a system must be in place. Such systems can include many nonsurgeon providers such as physical therapists and clinical officers. Braces can be made using local resources, but a mechanism for follow-up must exist to ensure that patients adhere to the bracing program, as the relapse rate may be as high as 70% when the brace is not worn. Regular follow-up also helps to identify the subset of patients who have a relapse, so that prompt treatment can be delivered. The results of numerous studies have indicated that, in contrast to extensive surgical procedures that often result in stiffness and overcorrection, patients treated by the Ponseti method have a mildly undercorrected foot that is mobile, functional, and has better results over the long term.

Nepal is a low-income country in Southeast Asia that has been politically un-stable for more than 15 years. While an active conflict between the Maoists and the government went on until 2008, the country has yet to achieve political sta-bility and a new constitution. The majority of the population is rural, with about 5% residing in the capital city of Kathmandu. Health service delivery is frag-mented, and numerous barriers exist to accessing health care, particularly in the more remote and rural areas. There has been no population-based strategy aimed at reducing the clubfoot burden.

The Hospital Rehabilitation Center for Disabled Children (HRDC) is a char-ity hospital in Nepal focusing exclusively on children's musculoskeletal problems. Founded in 1986, clubfoot deformity is the most common diagnosis it treats. The hospital typically sees more than 300 new cases of clubfoot per year, varying in age from infancy through adolescence. A significant number of new and resid-ual cases of clubfeet do not present for treatment. The strategy for treating club-feet in Nepal initially involved extensive soft-tissue releases, but in 2004 a treat-ment program using the Ponseti method was instituted.

Physiotherapists currently do the serial casting, and orthopaedic surgical resi-dents perform surgical procedures under the guidance of the attending staff. The braces are made in the hospital's workshop. Most patients require admission for the duration of their treatment because they often reside in remote villages throughout the country. A rehabilitation unit has been set up to cater to these patients. Following discharge, patients are seen for follow-up, either at the main hospital or more likely during one of the hospital's mobile camps closer to their homes. When the children return to their village, community-based reha-bilitation workers are available to monitor progress and solve any problems that develop, and occasionally the exchange or service of braces can be accomplished during one of the regional mobile camps. More than 2,500 clubfeet have been treated since 2004.

One challenge in Nepal was the realization that, although the Ponseti method was developed for infants, because of deficiencies in early diagnosis and referral, many children present after walking age. Initially it was unclear up to what age the technique might be successful. Despite limited data—but because of the great clubfoot burden—the HRDC team decided to use the technique for children up to the age of 6. The initial results were favorable and published in 2009. More than 80% of children were able to achieve a flat foot without the need for an ex-tensive surgical procedure. The team subsequently elected to extend the upper age for the Ponseti method to 10 years of age. The initial results in 55 children with a minimum two-year follow up are encouraging.

Implementing the Ponseti method in Nepal presented many challenges. Under ideal circumstances, an effective clubfoot system would involve several crucial components. The first would be screening for early case identification, ideally shortly after birth, as early treatment is easier and more effective. Perhaps midwives or others involved with maternal and child health care at the district level can be taught to make the diagnosis. Following diagnosis, referral must be made, as it is unlikely that clubfoot care will be available at the district level in LMICs in the foreseeable future. In Nepal, clubfoot care is focused at HRDC, a tertiary facility in the center of the country. While this focus initially made sense, a new method is being introduced, and the HRDC team must learn whether it is effective in their hands and well accepted by the patient population. Experience is gained, opinions form, and then—if successful—the challenge becomes how to scale up service delivery. Service delivery must be decentralized to address geographic barriers and also the financial costs of getting to and from the treatment center. Many patients have to travel extensive distances, often by foot, to get to the hospital. Given the absence of a functional public health system, it is difficult if not impossible financially and practically to set up regional satellite clinics throughout the country, although it might be possible in partnership with the government or other nongovernmental organizations with an interest in clubfoot care. The lack of a functional public health or district hospital system may represent a difficult challenge. Regional treatment centers are a more realistic alternative, and HRDC has recently developed eastern and western satellites in the towns of Itahari and Nepalgunj. Such satellites represent a positive step, but many patients in other areas of the country still lack access to clubfoot care. Training workshops are held every year to introduce orthopaedists and other practitioners to the method, but no data are yet available on whether other hospitals throughout the country have adopted the Ponseti method.

Evaluating the outcomes of the treatment program can be done at multiple levels: from the patient's perspective, from the provider's perspective, and at the level of the health system. Individual outcome measures include physical findings on bench exam or gait analysis, functional indices, and patient satisfaction. Function and patient satisfaction must be assessed with contextually relevant tools. Radiographic indices are not generally helpful and increase cost and radiation exposure. Infants treated effectively by the Ponseti method will have some mild residual deformities, but the feet are mobile because none of the joints have been disrupted surgically. Better mobility has been correlated with better functional outcomes, in comparison with extensive surgical releases that more often result in overcorrected feet as well as stiffness in violated joints. Studies of pedobarography indicate that patients treated effectively by the Ponseti method still put some excessive pressure on the outside of the midfoot or the foot's forepart, consistent with a mildly under corrected foot, but such compensation does not affect function.

Outcomes must also be assessed at the systems level because even the capacity to effectively correct the deformity at the tertiary center does not ensure that the correction will be maintained or that similar results can be achieved at satellite centers. Failure to adhere to a bracing program can result in relapse rates of up to 70%. It therefore becomes mandatory to ensure that a supply chain is intact to provide braces for the children, that adequate parental education is in place, and that the braces are comfortable to wear. Community-based follow-up is essential to address barriers to service delivery and for early identification of relapses.

There has been a global shift in the management of congenital clubfoot, and the minimally invasive Ponseti method now replaces the extensive soft-tissue release surgeries of the past. This technique is suitable for a "public health" approach to clubfoot care, as task shifting may be utilized successfully and common surgical procedures can be performed at peripheral health facilities. However, a "systems approach" will be required to scale up service delivery in LMICs by facilitating early diagnosis and prompt referral and treatment, as well as close monitoring within or close to the patient's home. Constant evaluation and monitoring will be required to identify and address barriers to adequate care, including maintenance of the supply chain and follow-up mechanisms, and to ensure that patient outcomes remain suitable for the community.

REFERENCES

Banskota B, Banskota AK, Regmi R, Shrestha OP, Rajbhandary T, Spiegel DA. The Ponseti method in untreated idiopathic clubfoot presenting between 5 and 10 years of age. *Bone Joint J.* 2013; 95-B: 1721–25.

Cooper DM, Dietz FR. Treatment of idiopathic clubfoot: a thirty-year follow-up note. *J Bone Joint Surg Am.* 1995; 77: 1477–89.

Dobbs MB, Nunley R, Schoenecker PL. Long-term follow-up of patients with clubfeet treated with extensive soft-tissue release. *J Bone Joint Surg Am.* 2006; 88: 986–96.

Jowett CR, Morcuende JA, Ramachandran M. Management of congenital talipes equinovarus using the Ponseti method: a systematic review. *J Bone Joint Surg Br.* 2011; 93: 1160–64.

Khan SA, Kumar A. Ponseti's manipulation in neglected clubfoot in children more than 7 years of age: a prospective evaluation of 25 feet with long-term follow-up. *J Pediatr Orthop B*. 2010; 19: 385–89.

Lourenco AF, Morcuende JA. Correction of neglected idiopathic clubfoot by the Ponseti method. *J Bone Joint Surg Br*. 2007; 89B: 378–81.

Ponseti IV. *Congenital Clubfoot: Fundamentals of Treatment*. New York: Oxford University Press; 1996.

Spiegel DA, Shrestha OP, Sitoula P, Rajbhandary T, Bijukachhe B, Banskota AK. Ponseti method for untreated idiopathic clubfeet in Nepalese patients from 1 to 6 years of age. *Clin Orthop Relat Res*. 2009; 467: 1164–70.

Tindall AJ, Steinlechner CWB, Lavy CBD, Mannion S, Mkandawire N. Results of manipulation of idiopathic clubfoot deformity in Malawi by orthopaedic clinical officers using the Ponseti method: a realistic alternative for the developing world? *J Pediatr Orthop*. 2005; 25: 627–29.

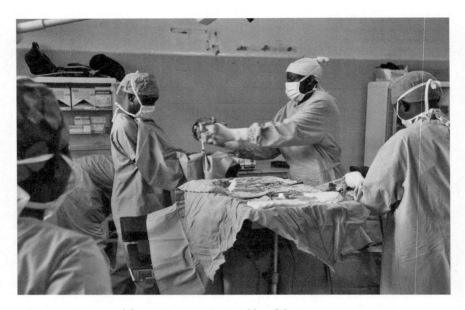

Figure 3.1. Cesarean delivery, Democratic Republic of the Congo.
Photo courtesy Chiels Liu

CHAPTER THREE

Women's Health

Access to Cesarean Sections in Ethiopia

LAUREN OWENS, MD, MPH, TIGISTU ADAMU ASHENGO,
MD, MPH, AND JEAN ANDERSON, MD

"She was brought in on a donkey cart." My response was a surprised "What?" She replied, "Yes, in the middle of the night, almost Christmas Eve. I was called to do an emergency C-section. It was pretty tough—ruptured uterus and the fetus was dead; the woman almost died herself. Luckily we were able to save her. But, yes, she arrived on a donkey cart." "Wait a second," I said, "back up. What exactly happened?"

It's a pretty common story in this region. For a woman to be considered a "real" woman, she must deliver her first child alone. This means once her contractions begin, she must go into the bush and deliver by herself. The typical case we see here is a 12- or 13-year-old girl, not really a grown woman, who got married, got pregnant, and went out to deliver. But she was too young. Her pelvis was not fully developed, or maybe it was but the fetus was in a breech position. She could not deliver. So what did she do? At what point did she decide to give up and seek help? After 12 hours? 24? Then, if she survived and did go back to her village, there was probably a long discussion. She's not a "real" woman, but her mother might have been able to convince her husband or father to get money to travel, to arrange transport, to go for a day or two over unpaved roads to the only medical facility in the district via donkey cart. Out here it is a pretty common story. But imagine how many don't even make it to the hospital.

It was a difficult conversation to have about the conditions in an isolated district hospital, but it underscored some of the pressing issues in women's health. Although women's health is an important component of the global health agenda, with Millennium Development Goal Number 5 specifically addressing maternal mortality, much more is needed. Better education as well as skilled birth attendants and midwives will certainly help, but sometimes only surgery—a cesarean section—will save a woman's life. To provide cesarean sections, however, health systems must have the necessary infrastructure, equipment, supplies, and skilled personnel.

Although the number of women dying in childbirth per year has dropped from 523,000 in 1990 to 289,000 in 2013, 90% of these deaths still occur in developing countries.

The subject of women's health encompasses much more than just deaths during childbirth. Other conditions specific to women that can benefit from improved surgical care include family planning procedures such as safe abortions and hormonal implants. Surgical care is also an imperative for the proper diagnosis, treatment, and palliation of breast, cervical, and ovarian cancers. In addition, women suffer from breast abscesses and other gynecologic conditions such as fibroids and prolapse—all conditions that can benefit from access to surgical care.

Cesarean section is one of the most commonly performed surgeries worldwide and is the most common major surgical procedure in sub-Saharan Africa. Health-care workers perform cesareans for a wide variety of reasons: obstructed labor, uterine rupture, hemorrhage, malpresentation (e.g., breech), previous cesarean, fetal distress, and abnormal placentation, among others. Bleeding (hemorrhage) is the leading cause of maternal mortality in low- to middle-income countries and is responsible for one-fifth to one-third of these deaths. Obstructed labor occurs in 5% of live births and 8% of births where a mother dies in childbirth, and it is the primary cause of an obstetric fistula. Access to cesarean section prevents considerable morbidity and mortality of both women and neonates. Cesarean section is one of the signal functions of comprehensive emergency obstetric care as defined by the World Health Organization (WHO). Furthermore, cost-effectiveness modeling data from countries with low rates of cesarean deliveries found this procedure to be highly cost-effective at $251 to $3,462 per disability-adjusted life year. According to the WHO, cesarean sections should represent 5%–15% of births, but rates in sub-Saharan Africa are only in the 1%–2% range. The rate of cesarean section tends to be inversely related to maternal mortality.

In Ethiopia, a country in sub-Saharan Africa with a population of over 73 million, the overall maternal mortality rate is 667 per 100,000 women. Maternal deaths account for 30% of all female deaths between the ages of 14 and 49. There are over 140,000 women with obstetric fistula in Ethiopia. The national cesarean section rate is 0.6%, and a large discrepancy exists according to socioeconomic status and access between urban and rural areas. In a review of Demographic and Health Surveys data from Ethiopia in 2000, cesarean sections occurred in 0% of deliveries within the poorest quintile and 3.24% of deliveries in the richest quintile. In addition, although 93% of births in Ethiopia occur in rural areas, only 69% of cesareans performed by nonphysician clinicians and 60% of cesareans performed by physicians were for women living in rural areas. Thus, although the entire country lacks sufficient access to cesarean sections, poorer women and women living in rural areas are even less likely to receive an indicated cesarean section when compared to their wealthier, urban-dwelling counterparts.

An insufficient number of cesarean sections are performed in Ethiopia for numerous reasons, and deficiencies are found in leadership and governance, communities, health-care facilities, and the health-care workforce. Until recently, Ethiopia had only four medical schools, but a push by the government has increased this number to 33. These facilities are new, however, and there are still few trained OB-GYNs. Physicians are generally poorly paid, and many leave the public sector for better-paying jobs with nongovernmental organizations, private practice in urban areas, or overseas. As of 2009, only 12% of deliveries occurred with an attending skilled health professional in a health facility. There are many potential reasons why, including urban versus rural residence; geography, distance, and lack of transportation; lack of knowledge and awareness of potential birth complications; cultural beliefs or lack of health-care decision-making ability; concerns about cost; and perceptions of poor quality of care or prior negative experiences in health facilities. Ethiopia has a vast and varied terrain with an inadequate road system; in rainy seasons, some roads may be impassable or destroyed by heavy rain. The average household's distance to a paved road is 11 km, and the average distance to public transport is at least 18 km. The cost of transport may be sufficient to delay a women's timely referral to facilities providing comprehensive emergency obstetric care.

In addition, the cost of the cesarean itself may place a heavy burden on families. The average fee for cesarean sections is $13 in government facilities and $155 in nongovernment facilities. In comparison, the annual per capita health expenditure is $19.21. Furthermore, the female literacy rate is only 38%, and only an estimated 50% of women participate in decisions related to their own health care. Health-care facilities, particularly in rural areas, may lack not only trained providers able to perform cesarean sections but also the necessary infrastructure, including dependable light sources, sterilization, surgical instruments, antibiotics, ability to provide anesthesia, and access to safe blood products.

An intervention to increase women's access to cesarean section needs to begin with an assessment of current policies; guidelines; community knowledge, beliefs, and practices; transportation infrastructure; pre- and in-service training, supervision, and mentoring; and human and material resources, capacity, referral systems, and quality. At the facility level, such an assessment should include availability of dependable water and electricity; equipment and essential drugs;

blood, surgical, and anesthesia products; nursing-provider competency; existing policies and guidelines; and management systems affecting care delivery. The results of this assessment will determine specific interventions. Once interventions are implemented, a plan for monitoring and evaluation as well as ongoing quality improvement are essential to track and improve outcomes.

A multifaceted approach is crucial in any program to improve access to cesarean section. In Ethiopia, a new cadre of midlevel health-care providers has been developed, and they are being trained to do cesarean sections. Although task shifting surgical procedures to nonphysician providers is controversial, this strategy can offer access to needed services when no trained surgeon is available. A recent meta-analysis of six nonrandomized controlled trials in over 16,000 women in low-resource settings found no significant differences in maternal or perinatal deaths when C-section outcomes were compared between clinical officers and physicians; however, wound infections and dehiscence were more likely to complicate cesarean sections performed by clinical officers.

A potential intervention requires both community and health-care facility components. At the community level, the initial assessment needs to provide information, education, and counseling about the benefits of delivery in a facility with a skilled provider and about warning signs of pregnancy-related complications. Men along with community and religious leaders must be consulted and involved. The community must be mobilized to help solve issues related to transportation to first-line facilities and to higher levels of care when needed. Input into current barriers to care and potential solutions are necessary. If possible, a representative community advisory board should be formed to give ongoing counsel.

At the health facility level, a team approach should be promoted, with each member of the health-care team empowered to actively participate in identifying barriers and in problem solving. The Surgical Safety Checklist developed under the WHO Safe Surgery Saves Lives Program should be adapted and implemented as a safety and quality improvement intervention. Use of a partogram is beneficial for all labors so that abnormal labor patterns can be identified as early as possible. If contractions are too weak or infrequent, oxytocin can be given to augment labor, potentially avoiding an unnecessary surgical intervention. The partogram is also a major way to diagnose obstructed labor, however, in which case timely initiation of cesarean section can prevent significant maternal and perinatal morbidity or mortality, including uterine rupture, development of an obstetric fistula, infection, and hemorrhage. Finally, if a cesarean section is needed but resources are not available on site, a referral system must be in place, including transportation to a higher level of care with appropriate communications with the facility.

An alternative and complementary approach to this problem is to focus directly on the low proportion of women who deliver with a skilled provider in a health-care facility. Lower rates of maternal and neonatal mortality and morbidity have been linked to giving birth in a health facility with the help of skilled medical personnel, and access to needed cesarean sections first requires access to a health-care facility. Studies in Ethiopia have shown that higher levels of delivery in a facility have been associated with higher levels of education with presumably greater levels of awareness of potential problems, greater exposure to mass media, and at least four antenatal visits. Increasing knowledge and awareness in the community through mass media campaigns, peer counseling at coffee ceremonies—common in social gatherings in Ethiopia—or the involvement of religious leaders are all examples of targeted interventions. At the same time, interventions with local health-care providers and in facilities to promote more respectful and high-quality patient-centered care are critical.

One intervention in Africa occurred in a partnership between the nongovernmental organization CARE and the Averting Maternal Death and Disability Program at Columbia University. Its goal was to improve access to emergency obstetric care (EmOC). Nine indicators comprise basic and comprehensive EmOC: intravenous antibiotics, anticonvulsants, uterotonics, manual extraction of the placenta, removal of retained products of conception, blood transfusion, basic neonatal resuscitation, operative vaginal delivery, and cesarean section.

Given the complexity of this issue, a multifaceted intervention was chosen. First, a needs assessment was performed that evaluated infrastructure, equipment, medications, policies, staff training, and regional health systems. Gathering baseline information before acting allowed for interventions targeting weaknesses in health-care delivery and made it possible to assess the effect of the intervention. Based on the infrastructure assessment, major renovations of water supply systems and two maternity hospitals were planned. The government agreed to provide support for a third hospital. Provision of equipment—particularly surgical equipment—was another priority. Protocols and guidelines for EmOC were developed with national partners. A midwife group trained local medical professionals. To improve record keeping, new obstetric registries were created, and key variables were targeted for improved data collection.

Finally, in a quality improvement effort, emergency response teams were created, and maternal death audits were introduced. Providers were trained in teams to aid in team building. Medical professionals formed supervision teams to assess improvement.

The case study, which began in 2000, was a longitudinal multifaceted effort. One Ethiopian hospital received extensive renovations to allow treatment of its large catchment area of two million people. The Ethiopian government supported hospital renovations carried out through this project. In addition, regional and national partners assisted with the design and evaluation of the following interventions. Professional societies assisted government partners and university training hospitals with financial and technical resources.

While creating new registers, study staff found multiple registers within hospitals and consolidated crucial data into a single, central register. Staff from the American College of Nurse Midwives trained local professionals in a skills curriculum. In turn, the local professionals carried out refresher trainings. In addition, a multidisciplinary team was trained in emergency obstetric care. Quality improvement efforts emphasized client-oriented and provider-efficient services. Teams that received training reflected on their work to improve quality. Maternal death reviews were used to evaluate causes contributing to poor outcomes. This process assisted staff in understanding and preventing root causes of maternal morbidity and mortality.

Intervention efficacy was assessed with qualitative and continuous quantitative evaluations. The baseline assessment found that some facilities reporting comprehensive EmOC capacity did not actually have that capacity. The cesarean section rate increased from 0.2% at baseline to 0.4% in 2004. The case fatality rate fell from 10.4% to 5.2% within the same time period, and the met need for EmOC increased from 2% to 4.5%. (The United Nations–recommended met need for EmOC services is 100%.) The proportion of births occurring in EmOC facilities increased from 1.6% to 2%.

Data collection occurred throughout the project. Revision of obstetric registers was part of the package of interventions, which allowed for better monitoring of outcomes related to cesarean section provision. In particular, the rate of cesarean section was a crucial data point for monitoring.

Because training providers were part of the intervention, assessing provider comfort with cesarean was another indicator of study efficacy. Other opportunities for monitoring include adverse outcomes related to lack of cesarean section. These data would include obstetric fistula, prolonged labor, and fetal death in utero.

Lack of access to cesarean section is a significant contributor to maternal and perinatal morbidity and mortality. Although the most common major surgical procedure in Africa, cesarean section occurs at rates far below WHO-recommended levels. The reasons why are multifactorial, as are the potential solutions, and both will vary by country and region. To address this issue effectively requires a multilayered approach in communities and health-care systems. Key determinants known to affect access to cesarean sections must be measured and monitored. Ultimately, access to cesarean sections and other needed services that help prevent women from dying in pregnancy is a measure of the worth assigned to women in society. The low status of women in some parts of the world is the greatest barrier of all. Mahmoud Fathalla, president of the International Federation of Gynecology and Obstetrics, said it best: "Women are not dying because of disease we cannot treat. They are dying because societies have yet to make the decision that their lives are worth saving."

REFERENCES

Alkire BC, Vincent JR, Burns CT, Metzler IS, Farmer PE, Meara JG. Obstructed labor and caesarean delivery: the cost and benefit of surgical intervention. *PLoS One.* 2012; 7(4): e34595.

Fesseha N, Getachew A, Hiluf M, Gebrehiwot Y, Bailey P. A national review of cesarean delivery in Ethiopia. *Int J Gynaecol Obstet.* 2011; 115(1): 106–11.

Gessessew A, Barnabas GA, Prata N, Weidert K. Task shifting and sharing in Tigray, Ethiopia, to achieve comprehensive emergency obstetric care. *Int J Gynaecol Obstet.* 2011; 113(1): 28–31.

Haynes AB, Weiser TG, Berry WR, et al. A surgical safety checklist to reduce morbidity and mortality in a global population. *N Engl J Med.* 2009; 360: 491–99.

Kayongo M, Rubardt M, Butera J, Abdullah M, Mboninyibuka D, Madili M. Making EmOC a reality—CARE's experiences in areas of high maternal mortality in Africa. *Int J Gynaecol Obstet.* 2006; 92(3): 308–19.

Reshamwalla S, Gobeze AA, Ghosh S, Grimes C, Lavy C. Snapshot of surgical activity in rural Ethiopia: is enough being done? *World J Surg.* 2012; 36(5): 1049–55.

Ronsmans C, Holtz S, Stanton C. Socioeconomic differentials in caesarean rates in developing countries: a retrospective analysis. *Lancet.* 2006; 368(9546): 1516–23.

Wilson A, Lissauer D, Thangaratinam S, Khan KS, MacArthur C, Coomarasamy A. A comparison of clinical officers with medical doctors on outcomes of caesarean section in the developing world: meta-analysis of controlled studies. *BMJ.* 2011; 342: d2600. doi:10.1136/bmj.d2600.

World Health Organization, United Nations Population Fund, UNICEF, Mailman School of Public Health. *Monitoring Emergency Obstetric Care.* Geneva: WHO Press; 2009. http://www.unfpa.org/webdav/site/global/shared/documents/publications/2009/obstetric_monitoring.pdf. Accessed June 20, 2014.

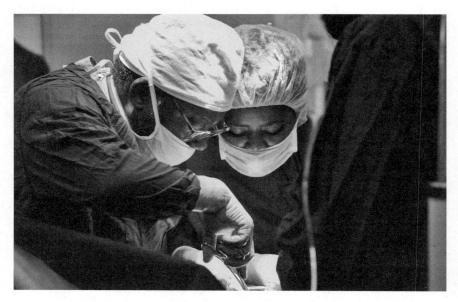

Figure 4.1. Lack of sufficient eye protection puts operating room staff at risk, Sierra Leone.
Photo courtesy Susan Hale Thomas

CHAPTER FOUR

HIV and Surgical Care

Improving Outcomes in Malawi

ANTHONY CHARLES, MD, MPH, FACS,
AND CARLOS VARELA, MD

"Doctor, we have none" was the terse response to the question "Why are you not wearing eye protection?" The nurse had seemed so cheery and helpful, but her attitude had instantly changed. Suddenly, my attempt to assist at a hospital in Africa was not going well.

Having taken for granted that all operating room personal would follow universal precautions—double-gloving (using two pairs of gloves), gowns, careful treatment of sharp instruments, and eye protection—seeing a scrub nurse without eye protection was a shock. In the United States, entering an operating room without proper eye protection, including glasses, goggles, or a visor, is not only unthinkable, it is illegal. The US Occupational Safety and Health Administration mandates wearing eye protection, and that is in a country with a relatively low prevalence of HIV. In a country with a high HIV prevalence, not using full protection was inconceivable.

At that moment the realization set in that, despite all the resources devoted to HIV prevention and treatment, one group was neglected and at risk of exposure to HIV: surgical health-care workers. Why was there not sufficient protective gear in operating rooms? Also, if surgical health-care workers were neglected, were there other conditions involving HIV and surgical care that were not receiving the attention they needed?

According to the World Health Organization, since the beginning of the HIV epidemic in 1985 until the end of 2011, almost 70 million people have been infected with HIV, and approximately 35 million people have died of AIDS. Worldwide, an estimated 0.8% of adults aged 15–49 are living with HIV in addition to 3.3 million children. Although the burden of the epidemic continues to vary considerably across countries and regions, sub-Saharan Africa accounts for 69% of persons living with HIV globally, with nearly one in every 20 adults (4.9%) infected.

HIV/AIDS is a medical disease that can be treated but not cured, and therefore prevention strategies are a priority. In communities and regions devastated by the epidemic, disease management is also mandatory. While significant efforts help to prevent HIV infection limit transmission and manage the disease, the knowledge of an individual's status is an important first step.

Malawi, a country in southeastern Africa with a population of 15 million, has felt a significant impact from the HIV epidemic. To care for the health of the population, voluntary counseling and testing were instituted early on the basis of WHO guidelines along with a universal opt-out testing policy for hospitalized inpatients. Near-universal availability of antiretroviral therapy (ART) is now available for HIV-positive patients, in large part because of funding and support from the US President's Emergency Plan for AIDS Relief.

A key step to overcome barriers to care is to obtain reliable estimates of the prevalence of HIV within a population. Such data help guide HIV prevention and management policies and assist with health-care delivery. In Malawi, the national prevalence of HIV decreased from 15% in 2000 to 11% in 2013. AIDS-associated mortality similarly decreased. These results arose from educational campaigns and the widespread availability of ART. Inadequate provision of HIV testing and counseling (HTC) and late ART initiation are two important factors preventing further reduction in HIV prevalence and incidence and the residual HIV-related mortality and morbidity. Despite ongoing efforts, HTC is not a routine part of care for surgical patients. Limited HIV testing in this population has resulted in a dearth of knowledge about the prevalence and epidemiology of HIV among surgical patients in southern Africa.

To obtain better estimates of the prevalence of HIV among surgical patients in Malawi, a study was conducted at a tertiary care government hospital in the capital city of Lilongwe. The study assessed the feasibility of conducting HTC using the existing public infrastructure and estimated the inpatient HIV prevalence in the setting of widespread ART availability. Data were also prospectively gathered on patients' clinical course and hospital outcome to investigate differences among HIV-positive and HIV-negative patients.

A universal opt-out HTC approach was used that was consistent with Malawi's national guidelines. Prior to the study, a trained counselor staffed the program, but HTC was done only when ordered by a clinician. To begin the study, all counselors were oriented to proper procedures and participated in sensitization activities designed to improve their knowledge and skills regarding opt-out HTC in surgical patients. During the study, counselors approached all patients admitted to the surgical wards and verified HIV and ART status. All patients with an unknown

HIV status or a negative HIV test result older than three months were offered HTC. The Malawi serial testing algorithm was followed using rapid testing: determine HIV-1/-2 as a screening test and Unigold HIV-1/-2 as a confirmatory test. Nonambulatory patients were offered bedside testing, which was the standard of care prior to the universal HTC implementation part of the study.

For the six-month period prior to universal opt-out HTC implementation, 270 patients were tested out of 2,606 total surgical admissions on the male (195 of 1,755) and female (75 of 851) adult surgical wards. Thirty-six of the tested patients (13%) were HIV-positive (10% of males, 21% of females).

During the six months of the study, 2,488 surgical admissions occurred. Fifty-three percent of admissions were elective, and 47% were for emergencies. Admitted patients' ages ranged from 13 to 102, with 68% being male. The most common indications for surgical admission were traumatic injuries and burns (28%), abdominal complaints (acute abdomen, bowel obstruction, hernia, nonacute abdominal pain; 19%), infections (abscess, infected wound, sepsis, cellulitis, osteomyelitis, septic joint, surgical site infection, pyomyositis; 12%), and tumors (known cancer, soft-tissue mass, other tumor; 9%).

HIV testing counselors approached 1,961, or 79%, of total admissions. Of the total approached, 8% were already known to be HIV-positive, and of those 83% were already on ART; for the others, 8% were known to be HIV-negative, and 1,651 of 1,961 (84%) had an unknown status and were offered testing.

Of those offered testing, 1,598 (97%) accepted, with only 53 patients (3%) refusing. The most common reason for refusal was not being prepared to know one's HIV status. No patients cited the bedside nature of testing as a reason for refusal. Of the newly tested patients, 136 of 1,598 (9%) were found to be HIV-positive. Thirteen (52%) of those were eligible for ART. Among all admitted patients, 1,598 (64%) received testing during their hospital admission, and 1,908 (77%) had a known HIV status by the time of discharge or death.

The prevalence of HIV among patients with a known status at discharge or death was 15% and was lower in males than females (14% vs. 18%). HIV-positive patients were also younger than HIV-negative patients (mean age 37 vs. 42), and HIV-positive males were slightly older than HIV-positive females (mean age 38 vs. 36). HIV prevalence in nontrauma patients was higher (16.4%) than in trauma patients (12.7%) when adjusted for sex and age. An admission diagnosis of an infection was specifically associated with an increased risk of being HIV-positive, as was a diagnosis of genital and anal warts or ulcers. However, HIV-positive patients were not more likely to require an operative intervention (incision and drainage, debridement, or amputation) when compared to HIV-negative patients. In fact, HIV-positive patients received surgical intervention less often overall than HIV-negative patients, and there was no significant association between HIV status and admission diagnosis, length of hospital stay, or mortality.

The study answered three important questions regarding HIV and surgical inpatients in a resource-limited setting in southern Africa. It showed that implementing universal HTC on surgical wards using existing infrastructure was feasible; that the estimated prevalence of HIV among adults on the surgical wards was 15%, a figure higher than the national estimate; and that there was no significant correlation of HIV status with increased mortality or length of stay.

In low- and middle-income countries, surgeons and surgical health-care workers have a unique opportunity to participate in HIV prevention and treatment. Occupational transmission of HIV to surgical health-care workers is a major concern for many providers, and the scarcity of adequate safety supplies poses a major problem. Another issue is the lack of reporting of occupational injuries or exposures. All health-care workers are encouraged to use universal precautions at all times, including double-gloving, using eye protection or face shields, and adopting a hands-free technique when working with sharp instruments or needles.

The frequency of cutaneous injuries caused by sharp items in surgical procedures is estimated to be between 1.5% and 15%, with an average risk of five injuries per 100 procedures. While the risk of exposure from a single-bore needlestick injury is 0.3%, a needlestick from a solid suture needle is significantly smaller, and no seroconversion following a solid suture needlestick has been reported. Needlestick injuries of health-care workers exposed to blood of patients on highly active antiretroviral therapy, or HAART, while low risk, because of the low or absent viral loads, do pose a possible risk for the transmission of drug-resistant HIV. The hands-free technique of handling sharp instruments and needles reduces occupational injuries and contamination by up to 60%.

Double-gloving substantially reduces the risk of contact with blood after a glove perforation. It is estimated that double-gloving reduces the amount of blood in a normal phlebotomy needle to less than 5%, effectively reducing the risk of transmission from 0.3% to 0.009%. Also, many glove perforations go unnoticed. The benefits of double-gloving far outweigh the perceived loss of tactile sensation and dexterity.

While a theoretical risk of surgeon-to-patient transmission exists, few cases have been documented. While the actual risk to a patient is minimal, debate continues about whether an HIV-positive surgeon should reveal their HIV status to all potential patients.

The risk of HIV transmission from patient to surgeon depends on the prevalence of HIV in the population served by the surgeon; frequency of accidental injuries with exposure to infected blood or body fluids; availability of HIV tests and postexposure prophylaxis in the institution in which the surgeon works; and, importantly, compliance of the surgeon to postexposure prophylaxis.

HIV continues to present significant challenges in the care of the patients, especially in low-resource settings. The use of HAART has led to an increase in the survival of HIV-positive patients, turning this previously fatal disease into a chronic one. As a result, malignancies, chronic illnesses, and other emerging surgical diseases present in these patients, posing challenges for health-care providers.

REFERENCES

Bennett NT, Howard RJ. Quantity of blood inoculated in a needlestick injury from suture needles. *J Am Coll Surg.* 1994; 178: 107–10.

Haac BE, Charles AG, Matoga M, Lacourse SM, Nonsa D, Hosseinipour M. HIV testing and epidemiology in a hospital-based surgical cohort in Malawi. *World J Surg.* 2013; 37(9): 2122–28.

Kerr HL, Stewart N, Pace A, Elsayed S. Sharps injury reporting amongst surgeons. *Ann R Coll Surg Engl.* 2009; 91(5): 430–32.

Malawi Ministry of Health. *Guidelines for HIV Testing and Counseling (HTC).* 3rd ed. Lilongwe: Malawi Ministry of Health; 2009.

Phillips EK, Owusu-Ofori A, Jagger J. Bloodborne pathogen exposure risk among surgeons in sub-Saharan Africa. *Infect Control Hosp Epidemiol.* 2007; 28(12): 1334–36.

WHO Global Health Observatory. HIV/AIDS. http://www.who.int/gho/hiv/en/. Accessed June 20, 2014.

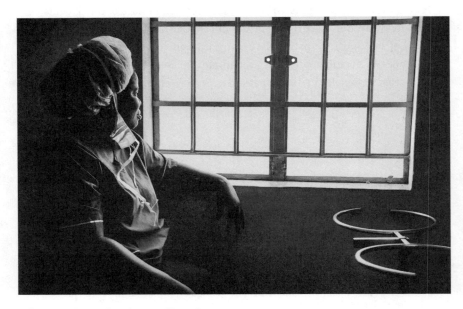

Figure 5.1. Operating theater, Sierra Leone.
Photo courtesy Susan Hale Thomas

CHAPTER FIVE

Cancer

Treatment in Low- and Middle-Income Countries

T. PETER KINGHAM, MD, AND OLUSEGUN I. ALATISE, MD

A woman presents with a large breast mass. The skin has broken down, the wound is infected, and she has large, firm lymph nodes in her armpit—there is little to offer but a simple palliative mastectomy to remove the source of the putrid drainage. A young man presents with difficulty swallowing, and a barium swallow shows inoperable esophageal cancer. There is no palliative care, so the best course is to send him home to die. A child presents with a large abdominal tumor. Clinically it appears to be a Wilms tumor. Surgery is performed and the tumor resected, but no chemotherapy is available. The surgeons hope the entire tumor was removed.

Three separate cases, all well advanced, all potentially curable. But the problem is that these patients lacked the education to seek treatment early; the health system lacked the ability to provide appropriate screening; and diagnostics were inadequate, with pathology results sometimes taking three months to be returned. Chemotherapy and radiation therapy were nonexistent, and surgical care, when available, was simply palliative or even too late to help.

Cancer is a rapidly growing clinical problem in low- to middle-income countries (LMICs) and in 2001 was the cause of death for an estimated 4.9 million people. Figures for the same year in high-income countries (HICs) were two million deaths. Over the next 30 years, an estimated 24 million people will die of cancer, and 17 million of them will be in LMICs.

There are several unique aspects to cancer care in LMICs. Up to one-quarter of these cancers are due to infections; however, the types of cancers that health-care providers see are changing, and there are now rising rates of colorectal, lung, breast, and prostate cancer. While mortality from cancer in HICs is 46%, cancer mortality rates are much higher—75%—in LMICs. The high case-fatality rate of cancer in LMICs led to a greater number of global deaths than AIDS, malaria, and tuberculosis combined. Reasons for the poorer outcomes for patients in LMICs include nonexistent oncology services, more advanced stages of presentation, lack of diagnostic and treatment options, poor compliance, and limited follow-up and palliative care.

As many cancer patients in LMICs present with late-stage disease, the mortality rate at hospitals is high. The association of high mortality from cancer at hospitals and within the medical establishment leads many patients to avoid going to the hospital at any point if they fear having a malignant tumor. Surgeons are commonly the first and only physicians to treat cancer patients in LMICs, so their experience and knowledge can help dispel rumors and increase trust in the medical establishment. Given their position, surgeons are important advocates for increased public awareness of cancer topics.

Obtaining a diagnosis is the first step in the management of patients with cancer. Pathologic evaluation of tumors is usually the primary mode of diagnosis. In tumors that are not amenable to biopsy, clinical judgment must help decide whether treatment is indicated. In locations without a pathologist, clinical judgment alone is sometimes used to make an initial diagnosis of cancer. Most patients in LMICs present with late-stage disease, often having large tumors, poor nutrition, and anemia. The clinical assessment must account for these symptoms and search for signs of local and distant spread of the cancer. For example, it is important to investigate for a cough or backache in patients with gastrointestinal malignancies, as they may suggest retroperitoneal, bone, or chest metastases. Just as trauma patients receive whole-body examinations, cancer patients should also receive a thorough head-to-toe examination. Lymph nodes, too, must be thoroughly assessed.

Staging patients with cancer in LMICs is often challenging owing to a lack of sophisticated technology and the reliance on more basic X-ray, ultrasound, and physical examination. CT scans are occasionally available in select centers, but the cost to the patient is often prohibitive. The first step in staging is determining the type of cancer that the patient has. Samples of a lesion can be obtained with a needle or with an open biopsy. Fine-needle aspiration cytology is commonly done in most LMICs because of its ease of use and low cost. The histologic findings must then be compared to the clinical scenario, as they must concur to ensure an accurate diagnosis. If the biopsy is inconsistent with the clinical scenario, then a repeat biopsy should be performed. Core biopsies can also be helpful, as they offer more diagnostic information when compared to fine-needle aspiration.

Surgery, chemotherapy, and radiation therapy are the three modes of treatment for cancer. Surgery is often the primary—and perhaps the only—treatment in LMICs because it is the only one of the three modalities that offers a potential cure. Surgery is often more available and cheaper than chemotherapy or radiation therapy. It is the primary modality for diagnosis, resection of primary tumors (and in select cases of metastatic tumors), and palliation.

Cancer surgery usually entails removal of the primary tumor with a margin of normal surrounding tissue and draining lymph nodes. The goal is to gain local control of the cancer and to prevent spread through direct extension and by vasculature seeding. Removal of the primary disease can also help to improve quality of life, especially in patients with large morbid tumors in their colon or breast. In HICs, organ-sparing procedures are common. In breast cancer cases, for example, lumpectomy with adjuvant radiation therapy is often performed. Owing to poor follow-up, limited therapeutics or a lack of sufficient patient education upon completion radiotherapy is often difficult to attain. Another requirement for breast-conserving surgery is the ability to perform a sentinel lymph node biopsy. It is difficult to translate this procedure common in HICs to LMICs because of a lack of local expertise, quality-assurance mechanisms, reliable pathology, and necessary equipment and supplies.

Adjunctive therapies for cancer include chemotherapy and radiotherapy. In LMICs, surgeons are often the only physicians prescribing chemotherapy to treat a cancer patient. This situation differs from HICs, where medical oncologists prescribe almost all chemotherapy regimens. Both drug availability and cost limit the use of chemotherapy in LMICs. Radiotherapy machines are also rare in most LMICs. Patients often have to travel long distances to reach a radiotherapy center, the costs of which—as well as of treatment—can be prohibitive. In addition, many of the machines are outdated, leading to high complication rates. Patients with cancers in LMICs are often seen at a late stage and are frequently younger than their counterparts in HICs. Surgery is one of the primary treatment options for both therapeutic and palliative care. Government legislation often limits opiate use, and access to hospice care is often not possible.

Although surgical care is recognized as an important aspect of providing care for patients with cancer, without additional resources, millions of patients will continue to die of treatable, curable disease.

REFERENCES

Adebamowo CA, Akarolo-Anthony S. Cancer in Africa: opportunities for collaborative research and training. *Afr J Med Med Sci.* 2009; 38 Suppl 2: 5–13.

Calle EE, Rodriguez C, Walker-Thurmond K, Thun MJ. Overweight, obesity, and mortality from cancer in a prospectively studied cohort of U.S. adults. *N Engl J Med.* 2003; 348(17): 1625–38.

Farmer P, Frenk J, Knaul FM, et al. Expansion of cancer care and control in countries of low and middle income: a call to action. *Lancet.* 2010; 376(9747): 1186–93.

Harper DM, Franco EL, Wheeler C, et al. Efficacy of a bivalent L1 virus-like particle vaccine in prevention of infection with human papillomavirus types 16 and 18 in young women: a randomised controlled trial. *Lancet.* 2004; 364(9447): 1757–65.

Lee CL, Hsieh KS, Ko YC. Trends in the incidence of hepatocellular carcinoma in boys and girls in Taiwan after large-scale hepatitis B vaccination. *Cancer Epidemiol Biomarkers Prev.* 2003; 12(1): 57–59.

Mellstedt H. Cancer initiatives in developing countries. *Ann Oncol.* 2006; 17 Suppl 8: viii24–31.

Parkin DM. The global health burden of infection-associated cancers in the year 2002. *Int J Cancer.* 2006; 118(12): 3030–44.

Parkin DM, Bray FI, Devesa SS. Cancer burden in the year 2000: the global picture. *Eur J Cancer.* 2001; 37 Suppl 8: S4-66.

Pisani P, Parkin DM, Ngelangel C, et al. Outcome of screening by clinical examination of the breast in a trial in the Philippines. *Int J Cancer.* 2006; 118(1): 149–54.

Sener SF, Grey N. The global burden of cancer. *J Surg Oncol.* 2005; 92(1): 1–3.

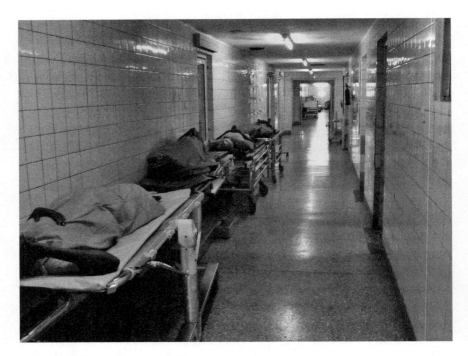

Figure 6.1. Waiting for surgery, Ghana.
Photo courtesy Mark Harris

CHAPTER SIX

Anesthesia

Educating Providers in Ghana

MARK HARRIS, MD, AND GABRIEL BOAKYE, MB, CHB

Health facilities in low- and middle-income countries (LMICs) frequently lack sufficient medical infrastructure, equipment, supplies, and adequately trained personnel. Performing safe operations with limited resources can make a surgeon feel like MacGyver. Instead of asking for the specific supplies and equipment, many surgeons ask for what is available and make do. A favorite device of mine is a cell phone with a built-in flashlight. During frequent power outages, it can be used to illuminate the operative field and allow an emergent procedure to be safely completed. Ideally, of course, there would be a constant power supply with a reliable backup, but often it is unavailable.

One important and also neglected component of providing surgical care in LMICs is the availability of anesthesia. While good at operating on patients who are asleep (anesthetized), surgeons cannot safely manage both monitoring an anesthetized patient and doing a procedure. In fact, modern surgery did not truly begin until anesthesia was invented in the 1870s. Before that, the sign of a good surgeon was speed rather than careful technique and knowledge—completing the procedure before the patient died from the stress of the procedure was paramount.

Although stories do exist of surgeons doing their own anesthesia, for many reasons this practice is not encouraged and is in fact dangerous. The patient must be monitored, anesthetic medications administered, and multiple adjustments made throughout the procedure. In addition, the care given after the operation is complete can dramatically affect the patient's recovery and the success of the procedure. Could the lack of anesthesia in developing countries be even more important than the lack of surgeons? Possibly.

Over the last 40 years, modern anesthesia practices in high-income countries (HICs) have led to a 40-fold improvement in perioperative care and patient safety. Over a similar timeline, anesthesia care in LMICs has remained underequipped, underfunded, and understaffed with persistently high morbidity and mortality.

When statistics are available from LMICs, anesthesia is usually in the top five causes of avoidable death, along with hypertension, hemorrhage, and sepsis. Most of the anesthesia-related deaths occur in rural hospitals, and 90% of them appear to be avoidable. Estimates of avoidable anesthesia-related mortality rates in LMICs are scarce and variable, ranging from one per 150 operations in Togo to one per 2,119 in Bangladesh. All the rates from LMICs are at least 10-fold greater than the one per 200,000 seen in HICs.

The Republic of Ghana is a small country in West Africa with a population of 25 million and only 15 physician anesthesiologists and 300 registered nurse anesthetists, which corresponds to 1.26 anesthesia providers per 100,000 people. Compare this figure to the United States, which has 24 anesthesia providers per 100,000 people. While 48% of Ghanaians live in rural areas, most of the anesthesia providers practice in urban centers.

Although many of the physician anesthesiologists in Ghana are heavily involved in the training of future providers, historically many anesthesia schools were one-teacher initiatives. Consequently, the increase in provider numbers has been slow. Nurse anesthetists in Ghana have a similar training pathway to their counterparts in the United States. With at least three years of postgraduate experience, nurses can apply to a nurse anesthesia-training program. The program lasts two years and includes a mix of classroom and operating room teaching, culminating in a six-month "apprenticeship."

In addition to physician and nurse anesthetists, there are many practitioners who are "trained on the job." These individuals range from high-school graduates formally trained over several years to anesthetist assistants who assume anesthetizing responsibilities when the previous anesthetist leaves the post or dies. With so few experienced practitioners, junior, relatively inexperienced personnel are often forced to perform procedures for which they are unprepared.

Opportunities for continuing medical education (CME) are also limited in Ghana. Access to up-to-date textbooks and journals is rare, and computer and Internet access, where it exists, is usually too slow for anything but the most basic functions. Before the International Anesthesia Education Forum (IAEF) Refresher Course was introduced, there were no formally recognized CME activities in Ghana.

Despite deficiencies of personnel, drugs, equipment, and infrastructure, many health facilities in LMICs perform high volumes of surgery, often with over 1,000 procedures per operating room per year, and over 2,000 procedures per year per anesthesiologist.

Until recently, there were no formal anesthesia residency programs in Ghana, primarily because of the low numbers of physician anesthesia providers available to provide teaching and mentorship for residents. In order to become an anesthesiologist, a physician had to spend several years in a residency in a HIC, most commonly in Europe. Ghanaian physicians, like many from LMICs who receive postgraduate training in Europe, frequently end up settling in those countries. Such émigré physicians state that the prime motivators for emigration are professional factors (e.g., specialist training, better facilities, and improved practice opportunities), with socioeconomic reasons such as security and finances playing a more important role in the decision to return home.

Gabriel Boakye is a Ghanaian physician who completed an anesthesia residency in Germany and returned to his homeland. He was instrumental in founding the first nurse anesthetist school in Ghana, at the Komfo Anokye Teaching Hospital (KATH), in 1987. He has directed the school since then, and by 2012 the school had contributed over 500 graduates to the nurse anesthetist pool in West Africa.

In the early 2000s a small group of anesthesiologists from the University of Utah started working in Ghana, initially participating in ophthalmic, orthopaedic, general, and urologic surgical missions. Realizing that Dr. Boakye could be helped by more than simple service projects, our team began teaching in the anesthetist training school. Thanks to a strong relationship with the anesthesia staff at KATH and other local hospitals and clinics, a need for CME for established practitioners was recognized.

The first Refresher Course was held in a small lecture room at KATH. Forty participants were expected, but 80 attended the course. Encouraged by the interest, the following year the course was held at a local hotel, enrolling over 100 participants. Since then, courses have averaged over 200 attendees per year. Most of the participants are nurse anesthetists from Ghana, but a significant number of the few Ghanaian physician anesthesiologists also attend. In recent years, attendees have included anesthesia providers from nearby countries, including Benin, Cameroon, Côte d'Ivoire, and Togo. As was always the intent, for the last five years the course has been organized entirely by Ghanaians, with our more formalized group of visitors (IAEF) providing invited speakers.

Since the first conference held in a hotel, a small fee has been charged to cover site rental and administrative costs—the host institution barely breaks even most years. Given that attendees (or often their regional health service) are financially engaged in the activity, charging a fee has contributed to an increased commitment to the educational endeavor. The Medical and Dental Council of Ghana recently certified the Refresher Course as the only approved source of CME credits for anesthetists within Ghana.

Various organizations have a multitude of projects ongoing in LMICs, such as long-term assistance with residency training, annual pediatric life support classes, and specific surgical techniques training. Where the Refresher Course project differs is in its transition to a course organized entirely by the LMIC providers. Although IAEF is still consulted on many aspects of these conferences, it is local faculty who run the courses. Local course organizers choose the topics, the speakers, and the format. Using IAEF academic experience where needed and the "exotic visiting professor" status as a draw for the first few years, once the annual conference is up and running, it is solely the property of the local group.

A Refresher Course is a series of lectures, seminars, or panels that reviews and updates a topic for those who have not kept abreast of developments in the field. The design of this course has many advantages over other formats (e.g., in–operating room teaching or small individual hospital teaching sessions):

1. In two days, a group of three people can update an audience of hundreds on a wide range of topics without interfering with direct patient care. This is a more efficient teaching method, and potentially safer than the ad hoc approach of in–operating room teaching. In addition, more technical subjects can be taught in smaller groups with hands-on stations, and "difficult case conferences" can highlight particular clinical issues. Such flexibility of format is advocated in adult learning theory.

2. Although hospital administrators may be welcoming and enthusiastic about an outside presence in their hospital, individual providers may not. The Refresher Course format avoids any perceived paternalism by a visiting practitioner or embarrassment of an established local practitioner. Local practitioners are invited to the course, and their attendance is voluntary and deliberate.

3. Providers from large and small as well as urban and rural institutions are encouraged to participate. Those from more isolated facilities often attend the meeting with particular patient-care issues in mind. A "difficult case conference" with their metropolitan colleagues can result in a beneficial level of professional communication that may seldom occur in a medically underserved country. Over the years we have seen many occasions in which practitioners from better-equipped regions donate equipment to their more deprived colleagues. They frequently state that they had no knowledge of their associates' need until they talked at the conference.

4. Hosting a Refresher Course is an opportunity for the institution to function as a regional education center. This role can serve as a catalyst for further educational endeavors and intraregion collaboration. For example, several institutions affiliated with KATH have initiated similar programs for physician assistants and trauma physicians.
5. There may be few possibilities in a medically underserved region for geographically discrete anesthesia practitioners to gather. A Refresher Course can serve as an occasion for networking, society meetings, and collaboration. For several years, The Ghana Association of Nurse Anesthetists has coordinated their regional meeting to coincide with the Refresher Course.

Adult learning theory suggests that an understanding of participants' educational needs is vital to a successful learning environment. In the resource-poor world there are topics of universal interest to anesthetists, including trauma management, obstetric anesthesia, pediatric anesthesia, and regional anesthesia. In addition, there are smaller topics that are of recurring appeal, such as preoperative assessment, sickle cell disease, and anesthetic implications of infectious disease. Having a relatively limited range of topics enables our course providers to develop pedagogical content knowledge, or a well-organized and adaptable understanding of both the content and learners' common conceptions and misconceptions. Clinical experience in the low-resource world ensures that lectures are relevant to the participants with their limited equipment, drugs, and medical infrastructure.

Increased in-country postgraduate training might help slow the medical "brain drain" from medically underserved nations. And in an environment with limited access to equipment and medications, robust, up-to-date knowledge of physiology, pharmacology, and anatomy are of the utmost importance—the buffer engendered by sophisticated monitors and fast-acting drugs must be replaced by a predictive wisdom.

As to the specifics of the IAEF process, once an invitation from a host institution is received, the first step is a general needs assessment, which enables IAEF to direct the curriculum by defining potential needs in knowledge base or skill set. An attempt is then made to gain an appreciation of the regional practitioner population, practitioner education, caseload, patient demography, and available medications and equipment. Frequently this information is limited and inaccurate.

The general needs assessment continues on the first day with the host. The team shadows anesthesia providers in the operating rooms to further understand their working conditions. In addition, practitioners are interviewed regarding their diagnosis and management of classic anesthesia emergencies (e.g., laryngospasm and bronchospasm). This process is similar in format to a chart-stimulated recall examination or checklist evaluation as advocated by the Accreditation Council for Graduate Medical Education and the American Board of Medical Specialties.

The Refresher Course is held on days two and three of the visit. The format of these days varies somewhat depending on the topics selected by the host institution, but the team consistently pursues the Socratic method, maximally engaging the audience in the learning process. Not only is this a recommended technique for adult learning, but also it was found to enable participants to better direct the program to meet their needs.

A Difficult Case Conference is held on the evening between the two meeting days. This format can engender beneficial intraregional discussion, and it can provide the team with great insight into the attendees' educational requirements. Attendees consistently cite this activity as a most vital component of the conference. On the final day of the visit, a debriefing session is held with the hosts. The team shares the results of the needs assessment, assisting the hosts in the direction of their own ongoing educational projects. The team also solicits feedback regarding the utility of the course, the popularity of the selected topics, the competence of the presenters, and the desirability of a return visit.

The International Anesthesia Education Forum constructed a website to serve as a place for ongoing discussion and education. Given the limited Internet service and browser capabilities in the developing world, the website has a simple format to optimize load times. The site incorporates a description of the faculty, including areas of expertise; a summary of courses, including stripped-down versions of some lectures; and contact information. The primary, long-term aim of the IAEF course is improved perioperative safety for surgical patients in LMICs. There are several difficulties in evaluating the success or otherwise of this goal:

1. Morbidity and mortality statistics are difficult to obtain in LMICs. The reliable record-keeping systems required to monitor such vital statistics are only now being implemented in a few of the more developed LMICs' health services.
2. The ability to discern and attribute causation to said morbidity and mortality is even more challenging, requiring highly trained pathologists, sophisticated root-cause committees, and an accepting medical community.

3. The multitude of humanitarian surgical missions, medical education endeavors, and equipment donations in any given year makes it almost impossible to determine which intervention (if any) resulted in the change (if any) in perioperative events.

Given this complexity, IAEF has chosen to assess a surrogate. IAEF believes that an appropriate, ongoing, and responsive continuing medical education program is an important contributor to patient safety. Most HICs currently insist on continuing education as part of medical licensure. Given this fact, the important assessment is whether the courses increase the knowledge of the attendees. Course attendees repeatedly state that they value the courses. But are the courses really achieving what they aim to? Preliminary results imply that they are, with attendees increasing their knowledge between pre- and postlecture tests. We are currently awaiting results on the six-month test of retention of this knowledge.

Whatever measure of success the project has achieved has been a result of its organic growth. Having no preconceived ideas, IAEF was able to avoid the distant, diffuse, dictatorial "planner" approach. Spending so much time in the operating rooms of LMICs enabled the team to observe first hand the specific issues and types of training in demand. More importantly, the team developed relationships that facilitated open and frank discussion whenever the endeavor faltered. Without such long-term engagement from partners on both sides of the income divide, a project will flounder, and it always seems to be the "helpers" from the HICs who complain the most acrimoniously.

Dobson states that "the problem with teachers is the same as with pulse oximeters—there aren't enough of them." The main principle of IAEF is to develop a true cooperative in which anesthesia professionals from all over the globe promote continuing education. In the long term, IAEF would endeavor to create a cadre of educators whose goal would be to teach the teachers, establishing self-sustaining regional centers of education with faculty who are willing and able to take a local leadership role in anesthesia education.

REFERENCES

Bainbridge D, Martin J, Arango M, Cheng D. Perioperative and anaesthetic-related mortality in developed and developing countries: a systematic review and meta-analysis. *Lancet.* 2012; 380(9847): 1075–81.

Dobson M. Training the trainers. *Anaesthesia.* 2007; 62 Suppl 1: 96–102.

Easterly W. *The White Man's Burden: Why the West's Efforts to Aid the Rest Have Done So Much Ill and So Little Good.* New York: Penguin; 2006.

Eastwood JB, Conroy RE, Naicker S, West PA, Tutt RC, Plange-Rhule J. Loss of health professionals from sub-Saharan Africa: the pivotal role of the UK. *Lancet.* 2005; 365: 1893–900.

Khan MU, Khan FA. Anaesthesia-related mortality in developing countries. *Anaesth Intensive Care.* 2006; 34(4): 523–24.

National Committee on Confidential Enquiries into Maternal Deaths. *Saving mothers 2008–2010: Fifth report on the Confidential Enquiries into Maternal Deaths in South Africa.* 2010. http://sanac.org.za/resources/cat_view/7-publications/9-reports.

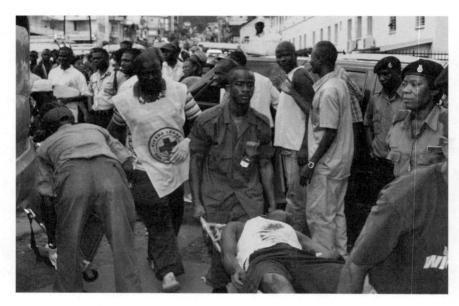

Figure 7.1. Mass casualty exercise, Sierra Leone.
Photo courtesy Glenna Gordon

CHAPTER SEVEN

Trauma

Implementing Trauma Registries in Tanzania

MARC DAKERMANDJI, MD, RESPICIOUS BONIFACE, MD,
MMED, MSC, HEATHER L. GILL, MD, MPH, TAREK RAZEK,
MD, AND DAN L. DECKELBAUM, MD, MPH

At first, her father refused to give permission to operate. "You can't do that type of operation here" was his rationale. There were only a few minutes available to convince him otherwise. His daughter, only 3 years old, had fallen from a balcony an hour earlier. She now lay in a hospital bed, paralyzed on one side and seizing on the other. Her right pupil was dilated. Clinically she had an epidural hematoma—a blood clot was rapidly expanding around her brain; within the hour, without an operation, she would be dead.

Technically, the father was correct. The hospital had no CT scanner and no neurosurgeons. His daughter needed holes drilled into her skull and the blood clot removed. In a high-income country (HIC), this would have been a medical emergency with a full team of specialized experts. But such specialists were not available in this case. Even so, without an operation, his daughter would certainly die. There was not much of a choice—ultimately, he consented to an operation.

Twenty minutes later, the little girl was asleep in the operating room, and the procedure began. A few moments later, holes were drilled in her skull, blood clots removed, and the nurse anesthetist reported that her vital signs had stabilized— she was improving. After the operation, the little girl was transferred to the small intensive care unit. The next morning she was awake and alert, and the following day she was transferred to a general ward. She recovered fully.

Although this story illustrates a classic "numerator" issue—treating a single patient, not a population—it began to spark my interest in trying to understand why donors and aid groups did not give greater support for surgical care. Even ministries of health seemed to ignore the massive need for surgical care for their populations.

As traumatic injuries and especially road traffic injuries increase throughout the world, improving surgical services for trauma care can play a preventive and therapeutic role. Adequately treating fractures and lacerations, which can be done even without the specialized knowledge of a surgeon or even a doctor, can prevent severe disabilities and even death. Major operations for conditions such as epidural hematomas or ruptured spleens can be lifesaving.

We need to look at traumatic injuries and surgical care from the standpoint of the population: millions are dying and hundreds of millions are permanently disabled from conditions that are preventable or treatable with surgical care. We need to examine the role that public health can play in improving surgical care for victims of trauma.

———————

The World Health Organization defines injury as "the physical damage when a human body is suddenly or briefly subjected to intolerable levels of energy." Throughout history, injuries have been thought of as unavoidable, as risks that go hand in hand with daily life. In the last few decades, however, injuries have been recognized as preventable events and have fallen under the umbrella of public health responsibilities. Concomitantly, there has been a growing concerted effort from the international public health and trauma care communities to mitigate the effect of trauma, primarily through innovative capacity-building interventions such as the development of trauma systems and trauma registries.

Trauma systems have been instrumental in achieving lower injury morbidity and mortality rates in North America. A trauma system is an entity that encompasses all aspects of patient care, namely, injury prevention and surveillance, prehospital care, hospital-based care, rehabilitation, and the meshing of hospitals within a comprehensive network. All of these components work in concert to provide an injured patient with the most appropriate level of care within the time frame that the patient's injuries require.

Trauma registries are key components of trauma systems, as they provide the critical data required for continual self-assessment and quality improvement. Modern trauma registries are exhaustive and intricate databases that document the acute phase of care of the trauma patient. Over the past 30 years, trauma registries have become an integral part of trauma systems in most HICs. They have been one of the driving forces behind significant improvements in both the prevention and the treatment of injuries. Unfortunately, these forms of reliable data collection are often unavailable in low- and middle-income countries (LMICs). A severe lack of resources and trained personnel constitutes a common roadblock to instituting sustainable injury surveillance, at least at the same degree of complexity as that of HICs.

A trauma registry is a database that is designed to collect a specific set of injury-related data, often during the acute phase of hospital care. Trauma registries have been shown to provide substantial benefits in a number of different areas. Their original purpose was to improve quality at the hospital level. Trauma registries collect data on variables linked to outcome measures in an ongoing and continuous fashion. By analyzing the data, hospitals can assess how their programs are functioning and assess for gaps in care. Ideally, a trauma registry collects uniform data describing individuals who meet specific inclusion criteria in which demographic, medical, injury severity, outcome, and other data are documented in an ongoing and systematic manner in order to serve predetermined purposes.

In HICs, trauma registries have become integral components of trauma systems at the hospital, regional, provincial, national, and even international levels. The first official civilian trauma registry as such was developed at Cook County Hospital in Chicago, Illinois, in 1969. This registry expanded quickly, and by 1971 it included data from 50 designated trauma centers across the state.

Over time, this outcome evaluation was scaled up to the national level. In 1982, researchers began work on the Major Trauma Outcome Study, where 139 centers across North America contributed to the database over a six-year span. Using the data as a benchmark, one could now estimate the expected mortality for a patient with any defined set of injuries, allowing hospitals and newly designed trauma programs to benchmark and compare their outcomes to the norm and to other similar programs. For the first time, data held hospitals to objective standards. As a result of trauma registries and valid data collection, countries are now able to closely and objectively monitor their trauma centers.

At a broader level, trauma registries can help influence public policy, identify specific gaps in injury epidemiology and call for the institution of education, prevention, and other policy measures to address these gaps. Registry data collected in Kampala, Uganda, for example, led the national government to declare injuries to be one of its top 10 health priorities. The data collected by trauma registries help orient decision making not only within local trauma systems but also at the national level.

Tanzania, like many other similar LMICs, has a significant injury burden. Between 1992 and 1998, trauma was second only to HIV/AIDS as a leading cause of death in this sub-Saharan nation. These data arise from the Adult Morbidity and Mortality Project conducted by the Tanzanian Ministry of Health as an initiative to produce cause-specific mortality data, performed using a community-based survey. Most available data in such LMICs are based on similar population surveys and extrapolations from mortuary and police reports. Although informative, they lack the accuracy and depth of information required to orient policy making. Consequently, an important precursor to improving the outcomes of trauma's heavy burden in Tanzania is to establish a more rigorous yet user-friendly data collection system adapted to such a resource-limited setting. Acknowledging both the urgency and challenge of establishing trauma registries in LMICs, more streamlined iterations of traditional registries have been developed.

In collaboration with the Injury Control Centre of Tanzania (ICC-T) and the Muhimbili Orthopaedic Institute (MOI) in Dar es Salaam, an urban Tanzanian trauma referral center and the nation's largest trauma-care facility, a streamlined trauma registry was established. The objectives were to establish the feasibility of implementing a trauma registry in a LMIC setting as well as to begin to define the characteristics of trauma patients arriving at MOI. The consequent gain of perspective provided a baseline level of data and offered a unique opportunity to employ and assess lessons learned from recently described initiatives in similar environments.

When planning a trauma registry in a resource-limited setting, it is important to understand the local context. The concept of contextualization is paramount because it may determine the success of implementing such a tool. In the LMIC setting, understanding the context implies working closely with local health-care leaders who will ultimately drive the execution and development of the program. At the request of the clinical leadership at MOI, the Centre for Global Surgery at the McGill University Health Centre formed a partnership with ICC-T to implement a trauma registry.

Using lessons learned from similar initiatives in Uganda, a streamlined and simplified data set was introduced. The data set was optimized to collect only relevant data, keeping it simple and user-friendly, so as not to overburden health-care providers working in already-busy centers. These were the key principles for effective implementation of the registry. This method as well as the tremendous local motivation to move forward allowed more significant widespread application to five peripheral hospitals across the country.

The widespread use of the registry generated impressive amounts of informative data on the many facets of the current state of trauma care in Tanzania, including striking information about who was actually arriving to the hospital or seeking care. Over 95% of trauma patients were presenting with injuries of low to moderate severity, meaning that only a small volume of patients with severe injuries was ever seen at a hospital. Many hypotheses have been generated, but the most likely scenario explaining this troubling disconnect between the known high incidence of trauma-related death in sub-Saharan Africa and the low numbers of sick patients arriving at the hospital was the presumed alarmingly high rate of prehospital deaths. Patients simply may not be going to the hospital to receive care. Moreover, the 5% that actually do arrive have a high 24-hour mortality rate, upward of 25%. This type of information may help draw attention to gaps within trauma systems, such as the need to improve prehospital care.

By defining the population of individuals who seek care—or, in the case of severely injured patients, those who actually survive to receive care—one can appreciate the maturity of a developing trauma system. While this sustainable hospital-based trauma registry has helped to identify the care-seeking trauma population in hospitals in Uganda and Tanzania, it has also demonstrated its remarkable ability to generate hypotheses regarding the current stage of development of the trauma system as a whole. An analysis of patient population patterns, injury-related characteristics, prehospital transport delays, and their associated outcomes allows us to better understand the areas that require focused capacity-building interventions.

Few studies performed in LMICs address the technical feasibility of implementing an injury surveillance protocol while also addressing the sustainability of the program. Sustainability in such settings often relies on the mixture of funding beyond the initial start-up support, trained personnel, material and technical support, and most importantly local commitment.

Successful injury surveillance data entry by understaffed, underpaid, and overworked clerks makes the Uganda and Tanzania initiatives noteworthy. Studies have elegantly shown the applicability of on-site computerized software-based data entry systems in developed settings. With increasing acceptability and receptiveness for the paper registries, the future use of electronic registries is becoming much more realistic. The benefit of electronic registries lies in live data collection and analysis as well as accurate capture and reliable storage of data. The greatest benefit of electronic registries is the scalability of implementation across centers able to support electronic formats, which in turn allows for benchmarking and comparisons within participating regions setting standards of care and quality assessment and improvement measures.

Tanzania, like many other LMICs in sub-Saharan Africa, is at an early stage in the development of its trauma system infrastructure. Thus it is precisely LMICs like Tanzania that stand to gain the most from the development of their respective trauma systems through the use of data generated by their trauma registries. As engagement and buy-in from local players increase, it will be paramount to create a unified database through regional organizations such as the West African College of Surgeons and the College of Surgeons of East, Central and Southern Africa.

The systematic application of such a standardized registry at the many echelons of care—from clinics and district hospitals to national referral hospitals throughout Tanzania and sub-Saharan Africa—will reinforce the ability to standardize expectations of patient outcomes and set performance benchmarks, providing the foundation for trauma system development and improvement in resource-limited settings.

REFERENCES

Barengo NC, Mkamba M, Mshana SM, Miettola, J. Road traffic accidents in Dar-es-Salaam, Tanzania during 1999 and 2001. *Int J Inj Contr Saf Promot.* 2006; 13(1): 52–54.

Centers for Disease Control and Prevention. Cause-specific adult mortality: evidence from community-based surveillance—selected sites, Tanzania, 1992–1998. *Morb Mortal Wkly Rep.* 2000; 49: 416–19.

Demyttenaere SV, Nansamba C, Nganwa A, Mutto M, Lett R, Razek T. Injury in Kampala, Uganda: 6 years later. *Can J Surg.* 2009; 52: E146–50.

Eisenberg, L. Global burden of disease. *Lancet.* 1997; 350: 143.

Kobusingye OC, Lett RR. Hospital-based trauma registries in Uganda. *J Trauma.* 2000; 48: 498–502.

McNicholl BP. The golden hour and prehospital trauma care. *Injury.* 1994; 25: 251–54.

Ministry of Health, The policy implications of Tanzania's mortality burden. Dar es Salaam, Tanzania; 2012: 1–56.

Mock C, Jurkovich GJ, nii-Amon-Kotei D, Arreola-Risa C, Maier RV. Trauma mortality patterns in three nations at different economic levels: implications for global trauma system development. *J Trauma.* 1998; 44: 804–12, discussion 812–14.

Mock C, Quansah R, Krishnan R, Arreola-Risa C, Rivara F. Strengthening the prevention and care of injuries worldwide. *Lancet* 2004; 363: 2172–79.

Schuurman N, Cinnamon J, Matzopoulos R, Fawcett V, Nicol A, Hameed SM. Collecting injury surveillance data in low- and middle-income countries: The Cape Town Trauma Registry pilot. *Glob Public Health* 2010; 6(8): 1–16.

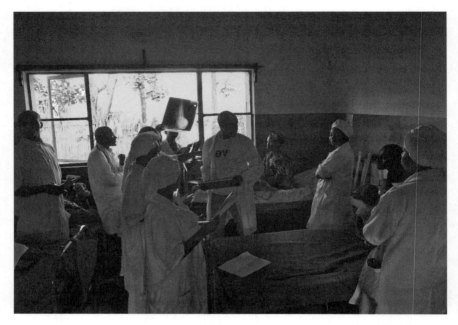

Figure 8.1. Ward rounds at a district hospital in the Democratic Republic of the Congo.
Photo courtesy Adam L. Kushner

CHAPTER EIGHT

Orthopaedics

The Institute for Global Orthopaedics and Traumatology

KUSHAL R. PATEL, MD, AND RICHARD A. GOSSELIN, MD, MPH

He was a teacher, 31 years old, and the father of three. A gunshot wound had shattered his femur (thigh bone). Such injuries usually heal by keeping the wound clean and restricting the patient to bed with traction for six weeks, but he was not so fortunate.

He developed a nonunion, where the ends of his femur did not fuse. His leg was no longer painful, but it flopped around and he could not walk. At a small rural district hospital in Africa with no X-ray machine and no orthopaedic surgeon, what were the options? A transfer to a specialist was not possible. One alternative was an amputation, but we thought there must be something better. I emailed orthopaedic experts from around the world for advice. The consensus was to operate, cleaning off the ends of the femur and stabilizing the leg so that the bones would have the possibility to grow together. There were no guarantees that the procedure would work, but we had no better options.

Luckily, the operation was a success and, except for a shortened leg that needed an elevated shoe, he could walk. It was not an ideal solution, but under the circumstances it was better than an amputation.

The lack of relatively simple orthopaedic care results in disabilities for millions of people around the world. Simple and safe procedures performed by surgeons, physicians, or even nonphysicians can treat many patients, and the personal and economic benefits are enormous.

Globally, an estimated 5.1 million people die each year from injuries sustained in road traffic crashes or as victims of violence, homicide, suicide, or war. Injuries account for 9.6% of the world's deaths and 11.2% of the global burden of disease. Ninety percent of these injury-related deaths occur in low- to middle-income countries (LMICs) where health-care infrastructure is lacking and health systems are unprepared to meet the burden. Injuries also account for 30% more deaths than malaria, tuberculosis, and HIV/AIDS combined. For every injury-related death, as many as 10 to 50 victims are left permanently disabled.

Although road traffic safety has emerged as a significant global public health challenge, limited efforts exist to improve overall injury care in LMICs. While preventative strategies are absolutely essential for reducing injuries and injury-related deaths, there will always be a need for health-care providers to manage and treat physical wounds. In hospitals in the United States as well as in LMICs, musculoskeletal injuries are common operative procedures; however, the burden of these injuries is much higher in LMICS.

A comparative study between San Francisco General Hospital (SFGH) in the United States and the Komfo Anokye Teaching Hospital (KATH) in Ghana showed a similar yearly volume of 2,132 versus 2,161 operative cases. On further analysis, KATH treated a disproportionately greater number of trauma cases (95% vs. 65%), severe fractures (29% vs. 15%), and infections (15% vs. 5%.) KATH also treated nearly twice as many open fractures and three times as many femoral fractures in comparison to SFGH.

In LMICs, the large burden of managing and treating musculoskeletal injuries often falls on a few trained health-care providers. In Ghana, there are only 0.10 orthopaedic surgeons per 100,000 population compared to 7.33 in the United States. Health facilities in LMICs also frequently lack adequate equipment and supplies to care for the injured. In addition to a lack of skilled health-care workers and resources, epidemiological data to document the magnitude of the problem of injuries in LMICs are largely nonexistent. Without these baseline data, implementation and monitoring of injury-related policies and projects are difficult. In an effort to improve injury care globally, The Institute for Global Orthopaedics and Traumatology (IGOT) was founded with a mission "to improve the care of underserved populations affected by orthopaedic trauma injuries through academic collaboration."

Various models to implement global health projects exist. The three most common are service-based organizations that rely on volunteers, nongovernmental organizations (NGOs) with professional and volunteer staff, and academic partnerships. Each model has its advantages and disadvantages. IGOT chose an academic partnership model to more readily form longitudinal and sustainable relationships on the basis of equity and mutual benefit. IGOT maximizes its resources by focusing on academic centers that help teach the teachers of tomorrow. An academic partnership also gives orthopaedic surgeons at partner sites access to institutional resources, mentorship, and career development. Long-term relationships allow

IGOT to truly understand the unique challenges that partner sites face and to better address their needs.

Modeling IGOT as a service-based volunteer organization would have duplicated other existing organizations, such as Operation Rainbow, and would not have allowed IGOT to better show how orthopaedic surgery is a cost-effective way to reduce the global burden of disease. Changing this perception is imperative if orthopaedic care is to ever be considered an important part of public health models in LMICs. Choosing to model IGOT as a NGO was a viable option, but by doing so the organization would have lost out on institutional resources and support from the University of California, San Francisco (UCSF). IGOT currently serves as a bridge between UCSF and partner sites.

The IGOT academic partnership is based on four pillars: Global Knowledge Exchange, Global Surgical Education, Global Research Initiative, and Global Advocacy and Leadership. The Global Knowledge Exchange program creates a two-way flow of knowledge between UCSF and IGOT's partner sites. IGOT facilitates travel for UCSF faculty and senior orthopaedic residents to teach at partner sites. Through the Global Surgical Education program, orthopaedic surgeons from partner sites are also able to come to UCSF as observers, as well as for courses and events that IGOT sponsors. The courses offered to IGOT partners teach relevant skills for resource-poor environments.

The Global Research Initiative at IGOT works with research institutions in LMICs that have important research questions but do not have the resources or skills to answer them. IGOT provides assistance and ongoing mentorship to partner institutions to build research capacity for critical issues such as adult and pediatric trauma, disaster management, cost-effectiveness, capacity building, and policy change.

To date, IGOT's Global Knowledge Exchange Program has facilitated the visits of more than 50 UCSF senior orthopaedic residents and faculty to partner institutions. These visits contribute through formal didactic lectures, impromptu teaching of theory, and operative skills and techniques. By exposing senior residents to orthopaedics in LMICs early in their careers, IGOT hopes to foster future domestic and international volunteerism, commitment to treating indigent patients, and help in addressing global burden of musculoskeletal conditions. Many residents have remained involved after completion of their training, and two are now on the executive board of Health Volunteers Overseas' Orthopaedic Overseas.

Every September since 2009, IGOT has held a three-day course known as the International Summit. The International Summit is the pearl of IGOT's Global

Surgical Education efforts. It consists of three courses: a precourse for residents on complex wound management, an International SMART (or Surgical Management and Reconstructive Training) course, and an International Research Symposium. The International Summit attracts more than 150 orthopaedic surgeons representing more than 15 different countries. IGOT's SMART course was developed in response to the large burden of open fractures with soft-tissue defects encountered in LMICs. These severe injuries are challenging to treat because skin and underlying tissue is lost, preventing surgeons from adequately closing the wound. These open injuries leave patients susceptible to infections that oftentimes can be treated only with amputations. In conjunction with plastic surgery faculty at UCSF and the University of Southern California, orthopaedic surgeons from LMICs are taught how to perform simple rotational flaps, which are skills that only plastic surgeons are typically taught. These rotational flaps allow for the treatment of soft-tissue defects associated with open fractures. In countries where plastic surgeons are unavailable, such skills are critical in reducing the morbidity of these severe injuries as well as preventing amputations. For countries in which plastic surgeons are available, these skills help avoid the delays that patients in LMICs often experience, improving patient outcomes.

In coordination with the Muhimbili Orthopaedic Institute (MOI) in Dar es Salaam, Tanzania, IGOT hosts an overseas trauma skills course. Over 100 surgeons from Tanzania and neighboring countries attend the annual three-day workshop, which covers the management of long-bone fractures with intramedullary nails, plates, and external fixation as well as the management of complex pelvic and acetabular injuries. Regional courses such as the one at MOI are not only more cost-effective but also much more accessible for orthopaedic surgeons from LMICs. Success of a course is dependent on the host institution's capacity, leadership, and political will. IGOT is also deeply involved in creating educational content for orthopaedic surgeons in LMICs. Those that have attended IGOT's International Summit are given access to step-by-step video instruction for performing rotational flaps learned during the SMART course. In addition, IGOT is developing an online research curriculum in response to partner requests for more formal didactics covering research topics.

The Global Research Initiative is based on the understanding that research is a key driver of a functional health-care system. LMICs need the ability to conduct quality research to assist decision makers in implementing effective health policies that are critical to the improvement of health-care systems. A recent survey of the orthopaedic literature found that less than 8% of published research originated from LMICs.

In addition to quantifying the musculoskeletal burden, IGOT undertakes research that supports the cost-effectiveness of orthopaedic care in reducing disease burden and that determines best practices in low-resource settings. With much of the research done in the management of orthopaedic injuries originating from HICs, where health-care providers have nearly limitless resources, little is known about how best to manage injuries in resource-poor environments. Since its inception, IGOT and its partners have published one to two peer-reviewed articles per month, ranging from studies that support the cost-effectiveness of orthopaedic care in LMICs to musculoskeletal disease burden determination.

The Global Orthopaedic Research Initiative also aims to foster research capacity in LMICs through education and mentorship. This aim is achieved by the annual International Research Symposium component of the International Summit. This meeting is a growing network of collaborators that provides longitudinal mentorship and supports an endowed research fellowship. During the research symposium, the fundamentals of research methodology and protocol design are taught. In addition to formal didactics, a small breakout workshop allows participants to develop their own research questions into research protocols. This "think tank" fosters a collaborative environment where ideas are discussed and has been the birthplace of many IGOT research projects.

Collecting data to evaluate outcomes of various IGOT endeavors continues to be a challenge, as many orthopaedic surgeons have neither the time nor resources to collect detailed data. For the SMART course, surveys are sent to participants one year after the course to assess use patterns. Survey results following the 2012 course showed that 32 participants (72.7% response rate) collectively performed 594 flaps, with 554 considered to be successful (93.3%). Of the successful flaps, 116 were believed to have prevented an amputation. Thirty-one of the 32 participants reported disseminating information to other colleagues or residents, with 28 other surgeons now performing rotational flaps. The skills and knowledge gained at this course by orthopaedic surgeons from LMICs were found to be quickly and extensively used in their home countries. IGOT believes strongly that this course represents a unique collaboration between orthopaedic and plastic surgeons to make a sustainable impact.

Comparing scholarly activity three years before and three years after the course will help evaluate IGOT's International Research Symposium. The number of abstracts, presentations, publications, and research proposals developed and accepted in each of the time intervals will determine that scholarly activity. The three-year time interval is included because of the inherent time required for research studies to take place and for manuscript preparation, submission, and acceptance processes. Results are yet to be determined, as the first International Research Symposium was held less than three years ago.

Looking forward, many hurdles remain, none more important than changing the perception of some in the global health community that orthopaedic care is not essential. Over the last decade, a growing body of research has supported surgery—in particular, orthopaedic surgery—as a cost-effective means of reducing the global burden of disease. The importance of preventing injuries cannot be understated, but it is essential to remember that even with the best preventive strategies, injuries will always occur. The global health community needs to work together to ensure that the capacity exists to treat these injuries regardless of whether they require surgery to prevent death and disability. IGOT remains focused on improving the care of musculoskeletal conditions and injuries globally through teaching, training, and research.

REFERENCES

Borse NN, Hyder AA. Call for more research on injury from the developing world: results of a bibliometric analysis. *Indian J Med Res.* 2009; 129: 321–26.

Brouillette MA, Kaiser SP, Konadu P, et al. Orthopedic surgery in the developing world: workforce and operative volumes in Ghana compared to those in the United States. *World J Surg.* 2014; 38(4): 849–57.

Davis SC, Diegel SW, Boundy RG. *Transportation Energy Data Book: Edition 31.* Washington, DC: Office of Energy Efficiency and Renewable Energy, US Department of Energy; 2012.

Debas HT, Gosselin RA, McCord C, Thind A. Surgery. In: Jamison D, Evans D, Alleyne G, et al., eds. *Disease Control Priorities in Developing Countries.* 2nd ed. New York: Oxford University Press; 2006.

Gosselin RA. The increasing burden of injuries in developing countries: direct and indirect consequences. *Tech Orthop.* 2009; 24: 230–32.

Lozano R, Naghavi M, Foreman K, et al. Global and regional mortality from 235 causes of death for 20 age groups in 1990 and 2010: a systematic analysis for the Global Burden of Disease Study 2010. *Lancet.* 2012; 380: 2095–128.

Mock C, Kobusingye O, Vu Anh L, et al. Human resources for the control of road traffic injury. *Bull World Health Organ.* 2005; 83: 294–300.

Mullan F. The metrics of the physician brain drain. *N Engl J Med.* 2005; 353: 1810–18.

Murray CJ, Vos T, Lozano R, et al. Disability-adjusted life years (DALYs) for 291 diseases and injuries in 21 regions, 1990–2010: a systematic analysis for the Global Burden of Disease Study 2010. *Lancet.* 2012; 380: 2197–223.

Nantulya VM, Reich MR. The neglected epidemic: road traffic injuries in developing countries. *BMJ.* 2002; 324: 1139–41.

World Health Organization. Injuries and violence: the facts. http://www.who.int/violence _injury_prevention/key_facts/en/. Accessed June 20, 2014.

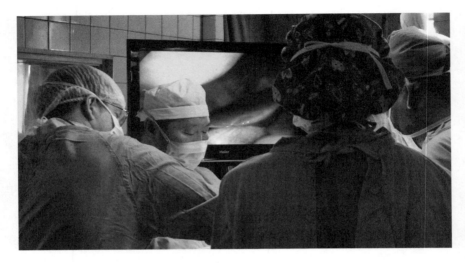

Figure 9.1. Laparoscopic surgery, Mongolia.
Photo courtesy Ray Price

CHAPTER NINE

Minimally Invasive Surgery

Challenges in Rural Mongolia

RAYMOND R. PRICE, MD, AND ORGOI SERGELEN, MD, PHD

Minimally invasive surgery—which includes endoscopic, laparoscopic, and robotic surgery—uses small cameras, fiberoptics, and other technology to help surgeons complete operations through small incisions. The advantages are shorter recovery times, decreased wound infections, and in many cases better outcomes. To safely undertake these procedures, however, surgeons and staff must be trained, specialized equipment and supplies must be on hand, and an uninterrupted power supply is essential. Given all the difficulties and limitations when planning surgical interventions in low- and middle-income countries (LMICs), I was skeptical that such techniques would be appropriate in low-resource settings.

Though I was initially opposed to using minimally invasive techniques in LMICs, over time my thoughts have changed. In 2004, I met a surgeon in Malawi who had worked at a mission hospital in Nepal. He had done the first laparoscopic procedures in that country and was also doing laparoscopic procedures in Malawi. He told me that it was possible to overcome some technical challenges. For example, CO_2 is needed to expand the abdomen, and and he was able to obtain canisters from a local Coca-Cola distributor. He was also able to cobble together a set of instruments from donated supplies. It worked and was safe. In Nepal, he initially charged patients who could pay high-income country (HIC) rates for laparoscopic procedures and used the proceeds to support the rest of the hospital and provide free care for the poor. I started to see that minimally invasive surgery was indeed possible in an LMIC.

Over time, after numerous discussions with LMIC- and US-based surgeons, I began to realize that minimally invasive surgery was not only appropriate for LMICs, but it was also really the treatment of choice. Certainly there was a lack of equipment, supplies, infrastructure, and training, but the patients in many LMICs are poor, being either daily workers or subsistence farmers. When they are sick and unable to work, they do not earn money. They rarely have sufficient savings, and their family can starve. Such people do not have the ability to spend a number of weeks recovering from an operation and need to be back to work as quickly as possible. I started to think that minimally invasive surgery was actually more appropriate in LMICs than HICs.

Introducing seemingly complex and resource intensive techniques in a LMIC does not at first make sense, but after examining the cost-effectiveness and the outcomes—quicker recovery, lower complication rates, and increased patient satisfaction—it seems that such interventions should be taken into consideration.

Recognizing that LMICs frequently need improved infrastructure development, the Dr. W. C. Swanson Family Foundation (SFF), a charitable nonprofit and non-denominational nongovernmental organization, established a medical warehouse program in 1998 that obtained surplus medical equipment and supplies and then distributed them to medical facilities in LMICs. Prior to distribution, medical re-pair biotechnicians would refurbish and recalibrate the equipment and then cer-tify that the items were in peak performance condition. In 2000, in an effort to make a tangible difference, the SFF decided to consolidate its efforts and adopt one country at a time. It first selected Mongolia.

Mongolia is a landlocked Asian country nestled between China and Siberia. It is the most sparsely populated country in the world, with a population of three million, yet covers a geographic area equal to that of France, Germany, Great Britain, and Italy. Vast rural areas coupled with extreme weather present signifi-cant obstacles, including inadequate roads and limited transportation options for patients in need. With 30% of the population still nomadic, access to health care for many in Mongolia is difficult.

While the Mongolian government provides national health insurance, signifi-cant deficiencies in infrastructure, supplies, equipment, and human resources exist at primary health-care facilities countrywide. Identifying the best possible ways for a nongovernmental organization to help improve health care required years of working in Mongolia, listening to the requests of Mongolian medical and surgical leaders, and discarding preconceived ideas about which interventions were possible and even best for the country.

The leadership of the SFF discussed many possible interventions, including developing hospital infrastructure by providing operating room tables, birthing beds, surgical instruments, X-ray machines, CT scanners, angiography machines, basic supplies, sterilization machines, diagnostic equipment, and computer support. Other options included providing medical or surgical training in basic emergency surgical care, basic surgical techniques, trauma care, obstetrics and gynecology, orthopaedics, oncology, and general medicine.

To help identify the most immediate critical infrastructure needs, represen-
tatives from the SFF met with political and health-care leaders in Mongolia to help
direct initial shipments of the highest-priority equipment. Numerous containers
with over $17 million of medical equipment and supplies were distributed to hos-
pitals in the capital city of Ulaanbaatar and many rural hospitals throughout the
country over 13 years. A basic set of open surgical equipment and instruments was
developed along with a program to upgrade all the rural hospitals in Mongolia
with this set.

But the impact to overall health care in Mongolia by simply targeting infrastructure development came into question. The SFF, along with local Mongolian
surgical leaders, decided that to harness the benefit of the improved infrastructure, they needed to provide education for the health-care providers. The SFF
began to organize various education teams of doctors, nurses, and biotechnicians to provide medical training and training for maintenance of the developing infrastructure.

In 2005 in Mongolia, like in most LMICs, injury was becoming recognized as
one of the leading causes of death and disability. Road traffic injuries were the
number one cause of death for males ages 20–24. That same year, the Fogarty
International Center of the National Institutes of Health convened a panel
of trauma and injury experts from the United States and LMICS who concluded
that trauma is particularly devastating in LMICs because of the lack of organized
and trained emergency medical services. Mongolia was no exception, with health-
care personnel who have no specific training in emergency procedures working in emergency departments and health facilities. Additionally, most health-
care facilities did not have a designated area to receive critical patients.
Emergency departments that did exist lacked the basic equipment and drugs vital
for emergency and trauma care.

Despite a need for improved trauma training, the local Mongolian health-care
providers did not have the same perception. To help address the need as viewed
by the SFF medical director and foundation chairman, the SFF organized a basic
trauma education team—including a trauma surgeon, anesthesiologist, operating room scrub technician, and biotechnician—to teach trauma care at the only
trauma hospital in Mongolia. The team prepared emergency and trauma lectures
that were based on preconceived needs, obtained the American College of Surgeons Trauma Evaluation and Management (TEAM) course, and then had the
lectures and course translated into Mongolian. A few months prior to the two-
week trauma training expedition, the SFF shipped to Mongolia a container of

surgical supplies appropriate for trauma evaluation in the emergency setting and for operative cases, which were then distributed to the National Orthopedic and Trauma Hospital of Mongolia. The SFF team was confident that they could help introduce projects to improve the standardization for the evaluation and management of the injured patient, leading to reduced adverse consequences of injury on health and society for all of Mongolia.

The local Mongolian trauma surgeons were cordial, and (with some struggle) were able to allot time for the trauma health-care providers, including students and residents, to attend the prepared lectures. The Mongolian medical student interest group seemed most responsive to the TEAM course lectures, while the senior Mongolian surgeons intimated that the information was too basic. The SFF trauma team operated with the local surgeons, but the senior faculty did not seem to think that they needed the suggestions of foreign surgeons. The local surgeons had significant operative trauma experience in this resource-limited environment and were confident that their care was not only adequate but also appropriate.

Basic modern trauma care in Mongolia was significantly lacking, however. There was no formal documentation of regular vital signs, the absence of initial evaluation and management guidelines led to significant missed life-threatening injuries, and operative procedures were antiquated. Although there was an urgent need for improved trauma care, recognition of the need by the local medical community was nonexistent, and initial and even early subsequent attempts for intervention were unsustainable.

During the 2005 trauma training expedition, the chief of surgery at the Health Sciences University of Mongolia (HSUM), Orgoi Sergelen, invited the SFF trauma team to the National Central Hospital of Mongolia (Hospital 1, the main academic teaching hospital in Mongolia) to see what they were doing with laparoscopic surgery. The team initially thought it would detract from their limited time to make a difference with trauma training at the trauma hospital, and that laparoscopy should not be a priority for a low-income country with such limited resources and training. With insistence from Dr. Sergelen, however, the team spent three days operating and meeting with surgeons at Hospital 1.

It was during these three days that one of the greatest learning experiences on a global surgery partnership began. Dr. Sergelen had just returned from a trip to the World Health Organization (WHO) in Geneva, Switzerland, where she presented data from a small study about laparoscopic and open cholecystectomy (gallbladder removal) in Mongolia, which she then presented to the SFF trauma education team. Gallbladder disease, she said, was extremely common in Mongolia. The second-most common cause for inpatient morbidity was from gastrointestinal diseases, with liver diseases, appendicitis, and gallbladder diseases being the three top causes. While laparoscopic cholecystectomy had been introduced into Mongolia in 1994, by 2005, only 2% of the gallbladders were being removed laparoscopically, and only in Ulaanbaatar.

The study performed by Dr. Sergelen compared open cholecystectomy ($n = 3{,}050$) with laparoscopic cholecystectomy ($n = 160$). She demonstrated that wound infection rates were nearly 10 times higher with open cholecystectomy compared with laparoscopic cholecystectomy (12.5% vs. 1.3%, respectively), and hospital stays were 10–20 times longer for open cholecystectomy (7–20 vs. 1–2 days, respectively). She indicated that while laparoscopic cholecystectomy had become the gold standard for gallbladder removal in HICs, the benefits of laparoscopic surgery (less pain, rapid recovery and return to work, decreased hospitalization, and minimal scaring) seemed to elude most LMICs, and it was probably even more critical for people in LMICs to receive these benefits. With its citizens living a hard life, not able to afford to be out of work for long periods of time, Dr. Sergelen said, Mongolia could not afford the time and cost of increased wound complications coupled with frequent dressing changes. Her final slide contained the most compelling plea: "Introduction and further development of laparoscopic surgery in Mongolian surgical practice is demanded!"

Having just finished two weeks working within the Mongolian health-care system and seeing first-hand the lack of supplies and limited financial support, the SFF team had serious reservations about teaching laparoscopic surgery in Mongolia. The WHO had felt similarly and turned down a similar request for assistance in teaching laparoscopy, believing that the introduction of new and more expensive technology might produce an additional strain on an already-tenuous medical system. How could laparoscopy be financially sustainable in this environment? How could adequate equipment be purchased and maintained? Would laparoscopy be safe in a country with an intermittent electrical supply? Would only the wealthy be able to access the benefits of laparoscopy, further widening the surgical care gap between the wealthy and the poor? Once trained in more modern surgical techniques, would surgeons flee to other countries in search of better employment opportunities? And would initiating short-term two-week trainings lead to increased intraoperative and postoperative complications? Did the surgical workforce have the sufficient knowledge and resources to not only safely perform minimally invasive surgery but also deal with the complications that could arise?

Despite the seeming inadvisability of teaching laparoscopy in Mongolia, Dr. Sergelen could only see its benefits for patients as well as the medical community. With persistent lobbying of the SFF team, Dr. Sergelen convinced the team to return to Mongolia to teach a basic laparoscopic cholecystectomy course at Hospital 1.

In preparation, during the subsequent year, the SFF team and Dr. Sergelen organized an initial basic laparoscopic course, including one day of didactic lectures followed by four days of hands-on training doing six laparoscopic cholecystectomies per day. The SFF education team included a multidisciplinary team of two surgeons, an anesthesiologist, a scrub nurse, a scrub technician, a biotechnician, a surgical resident for research and data collection, logistic and support team members, and multiple translators. Each member of the team was assigned to train their Mongolian counterpart about their specialty's specific role in making laparoscopy safe and sustainable in Mongolia. The medical warehouse obtained and prepared the laparoscopic equipment and shipped it to Mongolia months prior to the team's arrival. Advance teams reviewed and enhanced the electrical capability in the operating rooms and set up and tested the donated equipment a couple of weeks before the course. Dr. Sergelen invited surgeons from around the country to participate in the course. While the excitement for the training was palpable, each of the attendees wanted to have hands-on training, which significantly limited any hope for an intensive experience needed to safely impart new skills. At the same time, the SFF sent separate education teams to the National Cancer Hospital and to the Maternal and Children's Hospital to teach surgical oncology and obstetrics and gynecology, respectively, in an effort to train more standard open surgical techniques.

During the initial laparoscopic training in 2006, Dr. Sergelen asked whether the SFF would teach laparoscopy to the surgeons in Erdenet, one of the four designated regional diagnostic and referral centers, the next year. She also asked if the team could coordinate the laparoscopic course with a basic essential surgical program begun by the WHO. This request was initially flatly refused. Not only were the initial concerns raised about laparoscopic training in Mongolia relevant, but also the SFF had seen that teaching large groups of people could not impart adequate knowledge in a short period of time. And to take laparoscopy to rural Mongolia presented many more logistical problems.

So the SFF team returned home having agreed, or so they believed, to return and teach just a basic emergency and essential surgery course in Erdenet while also agreeing to attempt to teach basic laparoscopic cholecystectomy once more in the capital city. But to transfer skills adequately, the SFF required that only two surgeons per operating room would participate in the hands-on experience for the eight days of operative training, and the SFF limited each room to only three laparoscopic cholecystectomies per operating room per day. Unbeknownst to the

TABLE 9.1.
Contents of the Dr. W. C. Swanson Family Foundation Emergency,
Trauma, and Essential Surgery Course in Mongolia

Avoiding Common Bile Duct Injuries
Diagnosis and Treatment of Small-Bowel Obstruction
Appendicitis
Hernia
Use of Vital Signs in Inpatient Management of Trauma Patients
Stabilization and Transport of the Trauma Patient
Recognition and Treatment of Traumatic Shock
Management of Spleen, Liver, and Pancreas Trauma

SSF team, this type of training with rapid acquisitions of graduated skills was a new education model unfamiliar to the Mongolian surgeons. Their training traditionally consisted of many years of watching and having limited hands-on experience. So the concept of having surgeons experience a graduated skills training over a two-week period where they were expected to be able to perform the procedure independently before the SFF team returned home was totally new and exciting. At the time, the SFF also worried that this model might impart just enough comfort with new skills that could lead to increased complications, especially the dreaded common bile duct injury that requires major intra-abdominal reconstructive surgery. The SFF team prepared an emergency, trauma, and essential surgery (ETES) course, still holding on to the concept that basic surgical care was a higher priority for Mongolian surgeons (table 9.1).

But months before the SFF team returned to Mongolia, Dr. Sergelen lobbied passionately for the SFF team to also teach laparoscopy in Erdenet. Finally, relenting to the persistent lobbying, the SFF team agreed to teach laparoscopic cholecystectomy in addition to the ETES course in Erdenet.

Erdenet is the second-largest city in Mongolia, a town of 80,000 people, but the hospital serves as a Regional Diagnostic Referral and Treatment Center (RDRTC) for a much larger northern central area of Mongolia including nearly 300,000 people. Although the SFF team did not recognize it at the time, their agreement to help teach laparoscopic surgical techniques at Erdenet was the beginning of Dr. Sergelen's countrywide initiative to improve surgical care, and thereby health care, in Mongolia.

Dr. Sergelen invited doctors of all specialties from the Erdenet hospital along with surgeons and anesthesiologists from surrounding hospitals (some traveling 11 hours) to attend the didactic laparoscopic and ETES lectures. The SFF also created a sterile technique course that was well received. But there were only three surgeons from Erdenet who participated in the practical portion of the course,

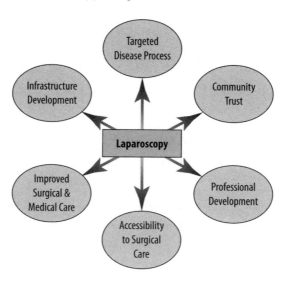

Figure 9.2. Laparoscopy: a mechanism to build sustainable surgical and medical care.

receiving enough experience to independently perform a laparoscopic cholecystectomy without assistance from the SFF educators. There were many unforeseen benefits to Dr. Sergelen's approach to involving health-care providers from the entire region and for including basic and laparoscopic training that helped create long-term sustainability (fig. 9.2).

Capacity for laparoscopic surgery was introduced to a RDRTC that improved access for people living in the northern provinces of Mongolia to modern surgical care. The training exposed the entire medical community in Erdenet to the benefits of laparoscopic surgery. Inviting care providers from smaller towns to attend the lectures, watch the surgery, and then witness the patient's rapid recovery helped convert the referring physicians to the benefits of this new procedure, leading to increased willingness to refer patients earlier in the course of their disease. The surrounding community was in awe as they watched their family members and friends recover from surgery so rapidly compared to the previous prolonged recovery times, creating a new trust amongst the people that they could receive good and safe health care locally.

All emergency, trauma, and essential surgical cases were additionally used as teaching cases during these two weeks, with the SFF team operating together with the local physicians. This endeavor provided a wealth of opportunities to address basic preoperative, intraoperative, and postoperative surgical care management. And rather than running into reluctance to change or adopt new methods, by providing a new and highly valued source of professional development, with the introduction of laparoscopy, a new level of trust and friendship developed between the local medical community and the external education teams, allowing for much broader training in basic surgical care and improvements in overall health care.

This new trust allowed the SFF teams to analyze critical infrastructure needs, which led to upgrading sterilization capability for open and laparoscopic surgery, introducing patient monitoring equipment in the operating rooms and intensive care units, and installing new anesthesia and cautery machines. Laparoscopy became the surrogate for improving surgical and medical care in Erdenet and the surrounding region.

Although Dr. Sergelen tried to articulate her plans for laparoscopy and ETES training in Mongolia during that initial presentation in 2005, it took the SFF team a couple of years to understand the true scope and possible benefits of her request. Dr. Sergelen essentially recommended a public health approach to treating gallbladder disease with minimally invasive surgery for the entire country of Mongolia while concomitantly improving basic surgical and medical care. The Ministry of Health identified an RDRTC for each of Mongolia's four geographical regions. Dr. Sergelen requested that the SFF teams, working with the local surgery experts, establish laparoscopic surgery and improve basic surgical care in each of these centers following the method used in Erdenet.

Before agreeing to such a process, the SFF team initiated a collaborative research project to study the safety of the SFF's short-term training method. The study compared the outcomes of patients receiving laparoscopic cholecystectomy from Erdenet, where surgeons had been trained with the SFF training course, to those of patients from hospitals in the capital city, where laparoscopy had been performed for many years. Surprisingly, complication rates were not different. Finally, converted to the benefits, safety, and efficacy of teaching laparoscopy in rural Mongolia as a formal initiative to improve health care in Mongolia, the SFF team committed to help establish laparoscopic capability in all four regions of the country (fig. 9.3).

Two additional RDRTCs were added, including major teaching facilities in the capital. Each site received two two-week training visits, and formal programs were created to help develop laparoscopic training capacity within the surgical residency program. These programs included the introduction of inanimate skills training modules. The Society of American Gastrointestinal and Endoscopic Surgeons (SAGES) kindly allowed the first four lectures from their Fundamentals of Laparoscopy course to be translated and used as part of the didactic curriculum. Then SAGES formally became a partner, sponsoring portions of the trainings from 2011

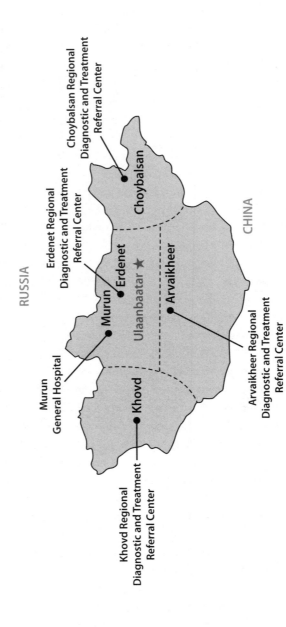

Figure 9.3. Laparoscopic training sites in Mongolia.

to 2013. Additionally, responding to the request of Dr. Sergelen and the surgical faculty at the HSUM, advanced laparoscopic training courses including minimally invasive surgical management of colorectal diseases and gastroesophageal diseases were taught in 2006, 2012, and 2013 to help expand the professors' laparoscopic capabilities.

A countrywide network of facilities with increasing capabilities concentrated resources regionally, which helped expand and utilize limited resources that can now be accessed by the entire Mongolian community. Many hospitals report that over 80% of gallbladders are removed laparoscopically, with very low morbidity and almost no mortality. Patients not only request but also are demanding the more minimally invasive approach.

Despite limited resources, the laparoscopic training program in Mongolia continues to stimulate growth of local capacity in laparoscopy and provide opportunities for other areas of health-care improvement. Following the advanced course in 2006, one surgeon participant has now completed 409 laparoscopic colectomies, mostly for stage T3 and T4 colon and rectal carcinomas. Another group of surgeons at the National Cancer Hospital designed their own technique for (and have recently completed 39) laparoscopic liver resections for hepatocellular carcinoma, the most common cancer in Mongolia. Mongolian surgical leaders now lead their own laparoscopic training teams, training additional surgeons and nurses at more sites around the country as hospitals begin to acquire their own equipment in a recently improving economy.

The many honors presented to SFF members from the Mongolian medical community, the Ministry of Health, and the president of Mongolia reflect the importance and success of Dr. Sergelen's vision for improving health care in Mongolia and the willingness of the SFF to listen and act upon her requests. Such recognition includes the bestowal of a professorship at the HSUM, honorary membership in the Mongolian Surgical Association, a medal of honor from the Ministry of Health, and the receipt of the Presidential Friendship Medal, the highest medal bestowed on a foreigner by the Mongolian president.

More importantly, the SFF's response to the many requests from Mongolia has assisted in developing other training programs, including orthopaedic spine surgery, surgical oncology, obstetrics and gynecology, general orthopaedics, internal medicine, and gastrointestinal and endoscopic training. Responding to the request for training in surgical oncology, simple introduction of self-retaining retractors, including Bookwalter and Omni retractors, led to a significant decrease in the backlog of liver cancer and stomach cancer patients, as the retractors allowed surgeons to operate more efficiently, tripling the volume of surgeries performed. Recent requests for training in cardiac, transplant, and pediatric surgery are undergoing evaluation.

Most interesting is the recent request for assistance in helping to improve trauma care in Mongolia, including the signing of a memorandum of understanding between the Health Development Department of Mongolia and the American College of Surgeons for initiation and countrywide training of the Advanced Trauma Life Support course for all doctors in Mongolia. A meeting facilitated by the medical director of the SFF under the direction of Dr. Sergelen included the vice minister of health, director of the health development department, leaders at the HSUM, director of emergency services for Mongolia, director of the ambulance service in Ulaanbaatar, and even the trauma surgical professors from the trauma hospital, and led to this new desire for improved trauma training in Mongolia.

People in HICs who desire to help improve the plight of those in LMICs often act upon preconceived ideas directed by the "obvious." But the concepts that seem so obvious from the HIC perspective may not be so obvious from the LMIC perspective. Conversely, the needs articulated by leaders in LMICs may seem to be totally inappropriate and even unobtainable from the outsider's perspective. Yet maybe, just maybe, listening and learning to understand the requests from our associates in LMICs will lead to greater dividends from initiatives directed by those who really know the local needs. While there may be many critical needs in any given area at the same time, successful, sustainable progress is likely to be achieved when local parties have helped identify the specific need and are passionate and motivated to find locally appropriate solutions.

REFERENCES

Gunsentsoodol B, Nachin B, Dashzeveg T. Surgery in Mongolia. *Arch Surg.* 2006; 141(12): 1254–57.

Hofman K, Primack A, Keusch G, Hrynkow S. Addressing the growing burden of trauma and injury in low- and middle-income countries. *Am J Public Health.* 2005; 95(1): 13–17.

Price R, Sergelen O, Unursaikhan C. Improving surgical care in Mongolia: a model for sustainable development. *World J Surg.* 2013; 37(7): 1492–99.

Sergelen O. Development of laparoscopic surgery in Mongolia. http://www.gfmer.ch /Medical_education_En/PGC_RH_2006/Reviews/pdf/Orgoi_laparoscopy_2006.pdf. Accessed July 21, 2014.

Spiegel DA, Choo S, Cherian M, et al. Quantifying surgical and anesthetic availability at primary health facilities in Mongolia. *World J Surg.* 2011; 35(2): 272–79.

Spogárd R, James M. Governance and democracy—the people's view: A global opinion poll. Washington, DC: Gallup; 1999. http://www.peace.ca/gallupmillenniumsurvey.htm.

Straub CM, Price RR, Matthews D, Handrahan DL, Sergelen D. Expanding laparoscopic cholecystectomy to rural Mongolia. *World J Surg.* 2011; 35(4): 751–59.

Vargas G, Price RR, Sergelen O, Lkhagvabayar B, Batcholuun P, Enkhamagalan T. A successful model for laparoscopic training in Mongolia. *Int Surg.* 2012; 97(4): 363–71.

Weiser TG, Regenbogen SE, Thompson KD, et al. An estimation of the global volume of surgery: a modelling strategy based on available data. *Lancet.* 2008; 372(9633): 139–44.

World Health Organization. *World Health Statistics 2011.* Geneva: 2011. http://en.wikipedia .org/wiki/List_of_countries_by_total_health_expenditure_%28PPP%29_per_capita.

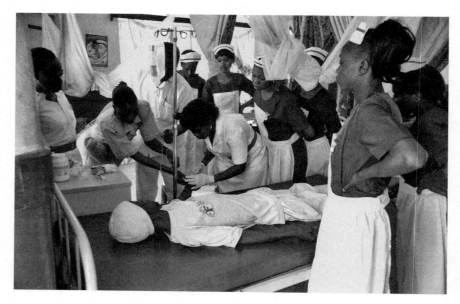

Figure 10.1. Teaching nursing students, Sierra Leone.
Photo courtesy Susan Hale Thomas

CHAPTER TEN

Surgical Process Improvement

Strategies to Combat Limitations in Ghana

IAIN ELLIOTT, BS, AMBER CALDWELL, BA, AND
RICHARD A. GOSSELIN, MD, MPH

The boy, only seven years old, had an infected wound. "How could that be?"

I was surprised, worried, and angry.

A few days earlier, he had climbed up the side of a passing vehicle. When he lost his balance and fell off, his leg got caught and snapped—resulting in an open tibia fracture. Luckily, he was quickly transported to our small district hospital. We rushed him to the operating room, thoroughly washed out and debrided the wound, bandaged it, and started antibiotics. I had no doubt it would heal. But something had gone wrong. The wound was infected.

I was new to this hospital. I had initially expressed surprise when the departing surgeon warned me during the handover that all dressing changes must be done in the operating room with copious amounts of hydrogen peroxide and iodine solution. I couldn't believe it. I had never heard of such a thing.

But something was seriously wrong. It wasn't just the boy's leg wound that was infected—all the postoperative wounds at our hospital were. To my utter shock and dismay, upon entering the project head's office and expressing my concern about the infection problem, I was told that "this is a dirty African hospital." I replied, "I've worked in 40 'dirty African hospitals,' and I've never seen this problem! When did it start?"

The project head explained that the postoperative infections had started three months prior, with the previous surgeon to blame. I now understood why he had resorted to doing all the dressing changes in the operating room, with what amounted to chemical sterilization. But none of this information made any sense.

"What else changed?" I asked. "No surgeon is that bad, something else must have changed."After a bit of hesitation, I was told, "Three months ago we also received a new expensive electric autoclave, but that couldn't be the problem. We checked it."

"What was done prior to this new autoclave?" I asked. The response was that instruments, drapes, gowns, and supplies were sterilized in an old-fashioned autoclave that was heated over a charcoal fire. "Good!" I said, "From now on we are going back to using the old method."

After returning to the old method of sterilization, the postoperative wound infection problem went away. Fortunately, the boy's fracture healed. A great deal of work was also needed to improve the overall functioning of the hospital, however; it was a complex and difficult task.

Health systems in low- to middle-income countries (LMICs) are frequently challenged with delivering quality care to large numbers of patients while facing resource limitations. Procuring additional resources is the typical solution to the dilemma of either treating more patients or improving care, yet increasing the efficiency of health-care delivery is a better long-term solution.

Inefficiencies in health-care delivery are not limited to LMICs. In the United States, health-care reform is driving change in the medical field, and hospital systems that do not address inefficiencies have difficulties maintaining financial viability. Inefficiencies in a health system also create conflict—health-care personnel know what is possible or recommended, which often differs from what can be provided. For example, appropriate treatment for an open tibia fracture is an initial washout and debridement with subsequent washouts and debridements performed every 48–72 hours until the wound is clean. But if a surgeon is unable to do a procedure because no operating room is available, the root causes of the problem must be identified. Process improvement is a methodology that can assist in identifying such problems.

Process improvement as defined by Alec Sharp and Patrick McDermott is "a systematic approach to help an organization optimize its underlying processes to achieve more efficient results." Multiple process improvement tools were initially designed for the manufacturing industry to maximize production efficiency. In health care, process improvement tools are useful to help care for more patients with the same resources, or to decrease the amount of resources required to treat each patient.

There are multiple process improvement strategies, all designed to increase the efficiency of a process. Six Sigma uses a rigorous statistical methodology to decrease errors and increase quality through the application of defining, measuring, analyzing, improving, and controlling. Another strategy, Lean, is designed to reduce waste in a system by simultaneously increasing flow and decreasing errors. Lean achieves increases in efficiency and decreases in waste production through continuously analyzing how work is performed, breaking it down to its individual components and determining which component actually moves the process toward a desired outcome. Plan Do Study Act involves a trial-and-error approach to process improvement through planning an intervention and a method to study it on a small scale, performing (doing) the intervention on a small scale, studying the effect of the intervention, and acting to either revise or implement the intervention more broadly (scaling up). Of use with all process improvement strategies and essential to the workflow of any system is Workflow Modeling, which helps to visually understand the complexities of a system and is necessary when determining how to analyze and intervene.

Surgical care relies on many pieces of "work" occurring in concert with one another to deliver a final product: a patient needing to recover from an operation or procedure. Overall care requires a functional operating room with surgeons, anesthesiologists, nurses, scrub techs and cleaners, anesthesia equipment, sterile tools, supplies such as sutures and gauze and implants, and a clean workspace; preoperative care; and postoperative care. The coordination of all of these components is extremely challenging, and a mismatch in preparedness or resource allocation can result in inefficiencies or the wasting of time and resources.

The complex nature of surgical care delivery means there are multiple stakeholders in any facility who must be included when initiating a project. One problem with redesigning any process is obtaining the support of all members of the team. To change a surgical care process, support is needed from heads of departments, faculty members, nurses, scrub techs, cleaning staff, and the facility administration. If lasting change is to take effect, all involved personnel must accept the plan.

To obtain a complete understanding of a process of care, all team members must be included from the beginning. Each department involved needs to be engaged, a leader or contact person identified, and then that individual interviewed and their work observed. The facility and resource problems that each person faces must be completely identified and understood. Communication barriers between and within departments must also be identified. Ultimately, all personnel involved in providing surgical care need to have their opinions heard, their work mapped, and their constraints and resource limitations understood. Without a complete understanding of the entire process from all points of view, progress is difficult and change does not last.

When the Department of Trauma and Orthopaedics leadership at the Komfo Anokye Teaching Hospital (KATH) in Kumasi, Ghana, sought to reduce the number of open tibia fracture infections at their facility, they used process improvement. With approximately 200 open tibia fractures a year treated at KATH, such cases are common and consume many resources. Even with the implementation of protocols for appropriate washout tasks and antibiotic administration, however, the number of infections had increased. Anecdotal evidence suggested that the major barrier to preventing these infections at KATH was the inability to provide ideal care because of an overwhelmed system. But what were the root causes of these infections? This question could only be answered by understanding the system as a whole, and the first step toward achieving that understanding was to examine each step by which open tibia fractures were treated.

Evidence from high-resource settings shows that serial washouts and delayed primary closure with the use of wound vacuum dressings is the gold standard for Gustilo type III open tibia fractures. The resources needed to meet this standard were deemed to be unavailable at KATH, not only because of the lack of wound vacuum technology and supplies, but also because of the inability to access sufficient operating room time.

Standard protocols for addressing open fractures are common in high-resource settings, and are used when possible in low-resource settings. At KATH, all patients with open fractures have an initial wound washout in the triage area, receive antibiotics as soon as possible, and undergo formal irrigation and debridement of the wound with an attempt to apply an external fixator within the first 24 hours of hospitalization. The importance of initial irrigation and debridement within six hours for open fractures is debatable, but strong agreement exists on the absolute need to accomplish this step within 24 hours. The Department of Accident and Emergency Medicine and the Department of Trauma and Orthopaedics at KATH were generally able to get patients into the operating room for their initial irrigation and debridement within 24 hours, and often within six hours. In addition, standard protocols were written and distributed to house officers who saw these patients as they arrived to the triage area. Unfortunately, wound infections continued to be high.

Ultimately, the leadership at KATH and the Institute of Global Orthopaedics and Traumatology initiated the Process Improvement Project for Operating Room Capacity and Patient Flow project as an initial approach to solve the problem of open tibia infections. To determine the best data collection points for a clinical study and where the system could be modified to increase efficiency, a workflow modeling approach was undertaken. It was hypothesized that a process map would help illustrate where improvements in the system could lead to lower infection rates and identify how these improvements could be measured.

The scope of the project at KATH included identifying all processes of care that affected patients presenting with open tibia fractures from the moment of arrival in the triage area until discharge from the hospital. The project was subsequently narrowed and concentrated on the care processes in the operating room, the perceived main bottleneck in the provision of ideal care.

After deciding to use process improvement, a choice of which strategy to implement was needed. The strong hierarchy at KATH made methodologies like Six Sigma and Lean difficult to use, as they require a change in management style and a handover of decision making to junior staff members. These strategies also require a commitment from the top decision makers of the hospital, as they affect all aspects of hospital operations, and were determined to be beyond the scope of the project.

Ultimately, a decision was made to focus on process mapping, similar to value stream mapping in Lean but with a focus on visualizing the complexity of the system in the form of a swim lane diagram. A swim lane diagram visually represents each person related to a process by a separate "lane." Boxes in the lanes represent tasks or pieces of "work"—something to do—that are necessary in the process. Arrows represent the path of the work in the process. The swim lane diagram identifies all actors (employees) of a given process, what their tasks are, how they interact with colleagues, and what inputs are necessary for certain steps to move forward. The swim lane diagram also helps identify areas of congestion and suggests how to simplify or manage the complexity. This visual map clearly and simply communicates how the individual actors' roles affect the system and how they influence each other. Once all the actors, tasks, and interactions are known, then the leadership team can more easily focus on identifying improvements using the existing infrastructure without seeking additional resources or personnel. This is a particularly important point for LMICs.

At KATH, the daily number of patients overwhelmed the system and the ability to get patients into the operating room, which presumably contributed to the high infection rate. For this project, the process mapping methodology was framed using the principles outlined in the second edition of *Workflow Modeling: Tools for Process Improvement and Application Development,* by Alec Sharp and Patrick McDermott. The process mapping methodology to improve the outcomes of open tibia fractures at KATH included:

1. Define the project's scope.
2. Identify key personnel.
3. Interview key personnel.
4. Develop a process map.
5. Shadow personnel to validate the process map.
6. Make recommendations for process modification.

A well-defined project scope is imperative. For this project, the leadership team defined the scope as improving operating room function to reduce open tibia infections. Once the scope is defined, key personnel critical to the functioning of the process are identified and interviewed. Data from the interviews are then used to create the swim lane diagram.

Figure 10.2 is an example of the swim lane diagram for this project (a small portion of the overall process map). Each lane represents a hospital employee and highlights their tasks in the process. For example, a specialist decides to operate and perform an elective procedure. He notifies a member or resident, who then writes an operating room list. The list then passes to the house officer, who distributes it to the operating room nurse and the anesthesiologist. All labs, X-rays,

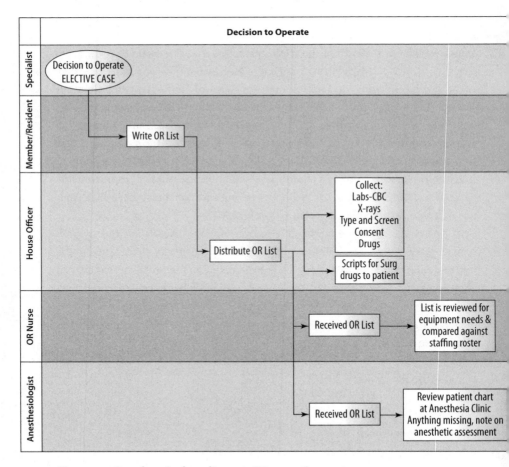

Figure 10.2. Sample swim lane diagram. OR, operating room.

consents, and drugs are double-checked, and the patient is prepared for the pro-cedure. If, for example, the pharmacy is on strike, the anesthetist must make sure the patient (or the patient's family) has prescriptions for the drugs necessary for the procedure. The operating room nurse receives the list and then checks on equipment availability and initiates processes to ensure that all is functioning. The anesthesiologist does a preoperative evaluation and notes if anything is missing.

The methodology used to design the map is dynamic and, if embraced, can serve as a practical and simple tool to advocate for and facilitate change in the sys-tem. Those involved in the process, at any level, can refer to the process map for clarification of workflow, contribute to feedback on improvement and solutions, and identify data collection points. Data can then be collected and framed as evi-dence to illustrate, in concrete terms, the limitations of an area of the map or sys-tem. This same approach can be used to advocate for particular solutions, using cost-effectiveness comparison and outcome measures as evidence. By systemati-cally approaching improvements in the workflow and documenting progress, the sustainability of the project is enhanced. The visual map also improves person-nel communication by identifying how each individual affects the workflow of others and the entire system.

The process improvement project at KATH identified several areas where im-provements in efficiency could be made. The problems all involved communica-tion breakdowns, and recommendations were primarily simple communication tools to intervene at critical points in the workflow. One recommendation was for an operating room white board to be placed in the center of the operative suite, to display all operations scheduled for the day. A second suggestion was for a tiered operative schedule, using a simple template to accommodate the time needed to sterilize the power supply when multiple cases required the use of a power drill. Of note, most recommendations had been made previously, but without the full support of the entire team, these recommendations had not been implemented or sustained over time.

A second site visit six months after the initial process improvement project measured the impact of the project and identified what changes the leadership team had made. Although most of the suggestions were pending administrative approval (particularly the allocation of an operating room manager), the changes that were adopted did have a positive impact on operating room efficiency. The surgical nurses took initiative to catalog and inventory all of the operative equip-ment and implemented a tray-labeling system to better identify equipment and to streamline the scheduling of cases on the basis of equipment availability. Also, a tiered scheduling system was adopted to better accommodate the addition of trauma add-on cases during the week. The department also reorganized the nurse's clinical duties and divided them into five teams instead of three. This reorganization allowed for a more even distribution of operative cases and increased the flexibility for emergency add-on operative cases. An incident book also documented case cancellations, equipment issues, and delays in operative efficiency, and was reviewed by the operating room leadership team once a month. In general, the leadership is optimistic about further improvements and committed to working on the project and adopting the principles and methodology of process improvement in other clinical areas.

The ultimate success of the Process Improvement Project for Operating Room Capacity and Patient Flow project will be determined by the continuous efforts of all stakeholders. Regular feedback will be needed, and leadership must be open to and accepting of all contributions from the staff, especially since those working closest to the problems often have the most realistic and feasible solutions.

When considering a partnership in a LMIC setting, process improvement with process mapping is valuable prior to initiating a project or clinical intervention (i.e., donations of supplies, clinical research, or change in practice.) These strategies and tools help illustrate where an intervention is most valuable and the effect on the system as a whole. From a public health perspective, process improvement contributes to the quality and sustainability of interventions, and is especially useful for projects that aim to improve surgical care in low-resource settings.

REFERENCES

Brouillette MA, Kaiser SP, Konadu P, Kumah-Ametepey RA, Aidoo AJ, Coughlin RC. Orthopedic surgery in the developing world: workforce and operative volumes in Ghana compared to those in the United States. *World J Surg.* 2014; 38(4): 849–57.

Carter PM, Desmond JS, Akanbobnaab C, et al. Optimizing clinical operations as part of a global emergency medicine initiative in Kumasi, Ghana: application of Lean Manufacturing principals to low resource health systems. *Acad Emerg Med.* 2012; 19(3): 338–47.

Nicolay CR, Purkayastha S, Greenhalgh A, et al. Systematic review of the application of quality improvement methodologies from the manufacturing industry to surgical healthcare. *Br J Surg.* 2012; 99: 324–35.

Sharp A, McDermott P. *Workflow Modeling: Tools for Process Improvement and Applications Development.* 2nd ed. Boston: Artech House; 2009.

Varkey P, Reller MK, Resar RK. Basics of quality improvement in health care. *Mayo Clin Proc.* 2007; 82: 735–39.

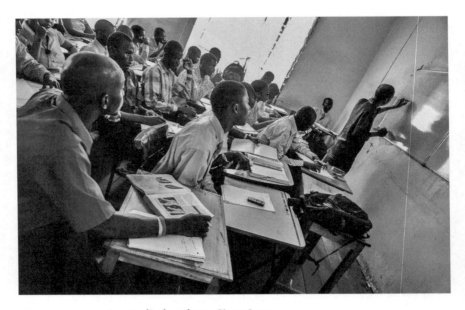

Figure 11.1. Lecturing medical students, Sierra Leone.
Photo courtesy Susan Hale Thomas

CHAPTER ELEVEN

Medical Student Education in Sub-Saharan Africa

JULIET S. OKOROH, MD, MPH, AND
BENEDICT C. NWOMEH, MD, MPH

A career workshop for medical students at the University of Liberia in Monrovia, Liberia, in the spring of 2012 highlighted the reasons for the surgical workforce crisis in sub-Saharan Africa. The goal of the workshop was to expose 100 medical students to opportunities for careers in surgical specialties. As the session opened, a show of hands revealed that only three students had considered a surgical career. Over the next six hours, the students heard several surgeons—including a general surgeon, a surgical oncologist, a pediatric surgeon, a thoracic surgeon, and others—describe their work. The workshop explored the frontiers of surgery and challenged the students to imagine the endless possibilities of new cures that the science and art of surgery could bring to millions around the world. At the end of the workshop, a show of hands revealed that 30 students now expressed an interest in surgery. While this experience reflects the reality that relatively few medical students show initial interest in surgical careers, it also shows that with a relatively brief exposure to surgical mentors, more of them will consider such careers.

There are 168 medical schools in sub-Saharan Africa, and one-third of them were founded after 1990. Many countries have responded to workforce challenges by investing in building new medical schools and expanding the class size. But many of these schools lack even basic infrastructure such as stable electricity, functioning latrines, and running water. Many teaching hospitals struggle to maintain basic sanitary conditions. There is often poor Internet access, and modern technologies for enhanced classroom, laboratory, and distance learning are absent, suboptimal, or poorly maintained. Even when available, some students are unfamiliar with the proper use of Internet resources for studying and searching the literature: in one study, nearly 40% of students reported having no training in computer skills. In a survey of 2,000 hospitals in sub-Saharan Africa, none had sufficient capacity to meet World Health Organization standards for "emergency and essential surgical care."

Several recent initiatives are poised to transform undergraduate medical education in Africa, including the US President's Emergency Plan for AIDS Relief (PEPFAR) and the Medical Education Partnership Initiative (MEPI) started in 2003 by US President George W. Bush. While PEPFAR's principal focus is to help save the lives of people suffering from HIV/AIDS around the world, its funding for various HIV-related initiatives has provided a major boost to funding medical education in the region. The National Institutes of Health (NIH)–sponsored MEPI grants provide funding to 13 medical schools in 12 countries that already receive PEPFAR support, with the goal to develop, expand, and enhance models of medical education. Both PEPFAR and MEPI have as overarching goals to increase the number of new health-care workers by 140,000, strengthen medical education systems, and build clinical and research capacity in Africa. By all accounts these programs have helped to strengthen curricula, upgrade Internet connectivity, increase access to current journal articles, build skills (simulation) labs, and incorporate distance learning. MEPI has also provided vital support for increasing expertise in neglected specialties, including surgery and cancer, by supporting the recruitment and retention of faculty.

Although MEPI has been the largest partnership for medical education in Africa—encompassing multiple US organizations such as the NIH, the Health Resources and Service Administration, the Centers for Disease Control, the Department of Defense, and the Agency for International Development—other partnerships between institutions in high-income countries (HICs) and African countries have also been strong in building the health systems of partner countries.

The global health community has long been concerned by the paucity of skilled health-care workers in sub-Saharan Africa. The health-care workforce challenge is particularly problematic in a region with 12% of the world's population and 24% of the global burden of disease, but only 3% of the skilled health-care workforce. The principal factor is the severely inadequate capacity to train the needed numbers of physicians and other health workers. The WHO estimates that at least 20 physicians per 100,000 population are required to provide basic health services. While all HICs have exceeded this target, many low- to middle-income countries are lagging behind, particularly countries in Africa. The United States has 240 physicians per 100,000 population, the United Kingdom 250, and France 340, yet sub-Saharan Africa has fewer than 18 (ranging from 60 in South Africa to two in Mozambique). Some countries have attempted to expand their training capacity, and indeed the number of both medical schools and enrollments has vastly increased. Of 100 medical schools, more than half were established in the past two decades alone, but not enough physicians are being trained to meet the demand. There are fewer than 10,000 graduates per year in the entire region compared to about 20,000 graduates per year in the United States. Through programs such as MEPI, there has been a vast increase in medical school enrollment in recent years.

A major contributing factor to the physician workforce crisis in sub-Saharan Africa is the so-called brain drain phenomenon. By some estimates, 22% of physicians from the region emigrate from the continent within five years of graduation, and the rate of emigration is increasing. Over the past 10 years, the rate of physician emigration from Nigeria and Ghana has increased by 50% (Ethiopia, >100%; Sudan, >200%). Liberia, one of the poorest countries in the region, has been the hardest hit, with more than three-quarters of its physicians having emigrated to the United States alone. Many of the émigré physicians are responding to domestic "push factors"—such as low wages, unstable working environments, and weak public health systems—and seek greener pastures in HICs. The migrant physicians are also partly drawn by "pull factors" from destination countries, including sophisticated recruitment strategies that target prospective migrants. Some HICs, such as the United States, have become chronically dependent on migrant workers, who make up one-quarter of their physician workforce and three-quarters of their primary care physicians. The loss of Africa's homegrown physicians has had a devastating effect on economic development but also medical education. For example, more than 60% of the locally trained physicians in Gambia have left the country. In addition, because many of the physicians who emigrate work in private clinics, when they leave, the lesser-skilled workers such as hires, technicians, cleaners, and security guards often lose their jobs. The fleeing physicians are often among the best and brightest in their countries; many were at the top of their class in medical school, and some were already teaching at a local medical school prior to leaving. Nearly all pursue additional specialist training in their destination HIC, but few eventually return to their home countries to help train the next generation of physicians. While many teach in medical schools abroad, two-thirds of faculty posts remain vacant in their home countries.

Using data from the Surgeons OverSeas Assessment of Surgical Need (SOSAS) surveys of Sierra Leone and Rwanda, it has been conservatively projected that 56 million people in sub-Saharan Africa suffer from conditions that are treatable by surgical intervention. Although there are limited data on the physician workforce

TABLE 11.1.
*Distribution of surgeons in seven African countries in comparison to
the United Kingdom and the United States*

Country	Surgeons (no.)	Surgeons per 100,000 population (no.)	Physicians per 100,000 population (no.)	Physicians who are surgeons (%)
Kenya	230	0.7	13.2	5.3
Malawi	9	0.1	1.1	9.1
Mozambique	35	0.2	2.4	8.3
South Africa	954	2.1	69.2	3.0
Tanzania	105	0.3	2.2	13.6
Uganda	63	0.4	4.7	6.5
United Kingdom	19,116	33.9	250	13.6
United States	135,808	43	240	18.0
Zambia	50	0.5	6.9	7.2

Source: Ameh E, Bickler S, Lakhoo K, et al. *Pediatric Surgery: A Comprehensive Text for Africa*. Seattle: Global Health; 2010. http://www.global-help.org/publications/books/book_pedsurgeryafrica.html#download.

and specialty distribution in the region, this burden of unmet need suggests a severe shortage of surgeons. Fewer than 10% of physicians in many African countries are surgeons, compared to 20% in the United States (table 11.1). By some estimates, the number of surgeons per population in the United States is 300 times that of the entire East African region. The shortage of surgeons across the entire region is even more pronounced for some subspecialties, particularly pediatric surgery.

At the root of this surgical workforce crisis is the lack of interest in surgical specialties by undergraduate medical students, as reflected in the career intentions of Liberian medical students. Decreasing interest of medical students in surgical residency training has been noted even in the United States. In one survey of medical students in Zaria, Nigeria, only 8% were interested in surgery prior to completing their surgery clerkship, mirroring the 7% preclerkship rate found in a survey of US students. In both cases, the postclerkship level of interest in surgical training significantly increased to 27.5% (Nigeria) and 40% (United States). Another survey from sub-Saharan Africa has confirmed that following the surgical clerkship up to one-third of the students expressed interest in surgical training. This might seem like a healthy level of interest in surgery, but anecdotal experience points to a sharp drop-off in the number that subsequently pursue surgical residencies or complete them, as reflected in table 11.1.

Why do so few medical students lack the desire to become surgeons in the first place? Does the overwhelming preference for infectious diseases over surgery among our class of Liberian students hold a clue? Some African surgeons have expressed frustration over losing some of their best students to specialties related to infectious diseases, such as internal medicine, pediatrics, and public health. They have speculated that massive funding of infectious diseases—such as HIV, malaria, and tuberculosis—by foreign governments and donor agencies has created a perverse incentive for trainees to pursue clinical and research careers related to these diseases. But these concerns have never been substantiated.

Surveys of medical students, including some from sub-Saharan Africa, cite the factors that are most influential in choosing a surgical specialty career, including faculty mentorship, length and perceived difficulty of training, clinical experience during rotation, participation in the operating room, interaction with residents, and lifestyle concerns, particularly duty hours. Anticipated income and other financial concerns are notably low among the most important factors that drive specialty interest.

Multiple surveys have revealed the critical role of mentorship by faculty, resident, and even student peers in helping to stimulate and sustain interest in surgical careers. Whether these surveys have been conducted in Western countries, sub-Saharan Africa, or other parts of the world, the vital role of surgical mentorship is preeminent. Below we discuss some ideas for increasing the capacity of the surgical workforce in countries of sub-Saharan Africa.

The few existing surgeons in Africa must take primary responsibility both for advocating increased resources for surgical care and stimulating more students to join their ranks. Our experience with conducting career development and mentorship workshops in several West African countries reveals that a relatively brief intervention can dramatically increase the interest in surgical careers. Frequently, individual mentorship of students by surgical faculty is lacking, and the students' experience during their surgical clerkships can be improved. In one survey, only 22% rated the overall quality of their surgery clerkship as excellent. The major suggestions for improving the clerkship quality included (1) more direct involvement in patient care and (2) more direct faculty–student interaction. These tangible measures are within the control of the surgical faculty, who should be more welcoming of students needing guidance and advice on career issues. Visiting surgeons on "medical missions" from other countries should consider sharing ideas with local faculty on best practices for student mentorship. Visiting medical students should share ideas with their local peers on peer mentorship activities, such as the role of surgical interest groups. The global surgery community should refocus efforts on training, faculty development, and capacity building, which will likely produce more lasting benefits than itinerant surgical operations.

Presumably, if we can convince everyone how important it is to train more surgeons, society will demand more surgeons, and more students will rise to the challenge. But few people in the countries of sub-Saharan Africa actually consider surgical care to be a vital need. We now know from available data that 56 million people in these countries need surgery today, but local officials, policymakers, the public, and even the medical community are not paying attention to this dire situation. Data on the burden of surgical diseases and surgical capacity surveys are welcome, and more are needed. These data need to be disseminated not just in elite medical journals but also in local journals, local medical conferences, and local media, and should be brought up in discussions with local officials, nongovernmental organizations, and other stakeholders.

So, we finally get students interested in surgery and the faculty line up to provide mentorship, but where are the training posts? There are still an estimated 56 million people waiting for surgery in sub-Saharan Africa, and though more surgeons are trained, are there real jobs awaiting them? Will there be operating theaters and other facilities for them to perform their jobs? Will there be job satisfaction? These are among the most perplexing questions.

Overall, there is little policy coordination between medical schools and ministries of health, education, and finance in many sub-Saharan African countries. This has not only budgetary consequences for funding medical education but also implications for health systems and human resource development. Even with such desperate need for physicians, many recent medical graduates remain unemployed for some time after graduation or take jobs unrelated to their training. Providing employment for surgeons and other physicians and infrastructural development is a task suited primarily for the individual governments.

With so much unmet need for surgical care in sub-Saharan Africa, the most effective and sustainable solution will come from efforts to develop local capacity in terms of personnel, health systems, equipment, and infrastructure. For the global surgery community, the main focus should be on how to train adequate numbers of African surgeons, and thus a planned obsolescence of "medical missions." If we are to achieve our goal of adequate surgical care, we must plan for the day when medical missions are obsolete, which can only be achieved by increasing local capacity. To achieve this goal, there must be a strong undergraduate medical education system, with robust curriculum, expanded capacity, adequate facilities, and high-quality faculty. For the few surgeons already in the trenches, their vital role must be in modeling skillful and compassionate care, and providing mentorship to the next generation that will take their place.

REFERENCES

Chen C, Buch E, Wassermann T, et al. A survey of sub-Saharan African medical schools. *Hum Resour Health.* 2012; 10: 4.

Ekenze SO, Ugwumba FO, Obi UM, Ekenze OS. Undergraduate surgery clerkship and the choice of surgery as a career: perspective from a developing country. *World J Surg.* 2013; 37(9): 2094–100.

Makama JG, Ameh EA. Does general surgery clerkship make a future career in surgery more appealing to medical students? *Afr Health Sci.* 2010; 10(3): 292–96.

O'Herrin JK, Lewis BJ, Rikkers LF, Chen H. Why do students choose careers in surgery? *J Surg Res.* 2004; 119(2): 124–29.

Tankwanchi AB, Ozden C, Vermund SH. Physician emigration from sub-Saharan Africa to the United States: analysis of the 2011 AMA physician masterfile. *PLoS Med.* 2013; 10(9): e1001513.

Taylor AL, Hwenda L, Larsen BI, Daulaire N. Stemming the brain drain—a WHO global code of practice on international recruitment of health personnel. *N Engl J Med.* 2011; 365(25): 2348–51.

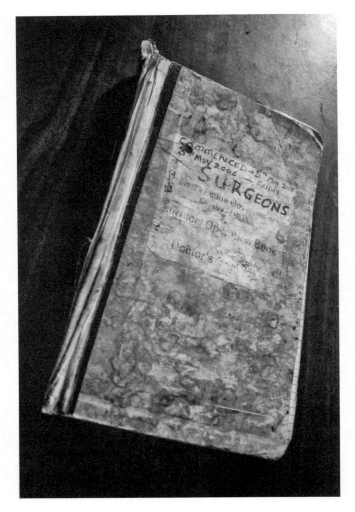

Figure C.1. Operating room logbook, Sierra Leone.
Photo courtesy Susan Hale Thomas

Conclusion

ADAM L. KUSHNER, MD, MPH, FACS, AND
EVAN G. WONG, MD, MPH

Access to surgical care is vital for good health care and integral to achieving a functioning health system. Too often in low- and middle-income countries (LMICs), wage earners die from injuries or preventable conditions such as obstructed hernias; children are permanently disabled without proper clubfoot or fracture management; and women die in childbirth or develop an obstetric fistula because of the lack of a cesarean section. Surgical conditions resulting from HIV, tuberculosis, cancer, and other noncommunicable diseases are all too common. To the frustration of many stakeholders, surgical care has been relatively absent from the public health and global health agendas.

In the course of putting together this book, the contributors were able to reflect on decades of global surgery experience, as illustrated in the vignettes and case studies from multiple LMICs in Africa and Asia. The stories demonstrate the reality for millions of patients and highlight conditions that are almost unimaginable in high-income countries (HICs).

The contributions to this book cover a broad range of topics that illustrate the varied nature of surgical care. Global surgery and surgical care are not limited to a single intervention or disease. Surgical care is needed for men and women, the old and the young. Surgical care cuts across disease silos and is important in treating patients with many conditions that can result from trauma, cancer, and even HIV, tuberculosis, and diabetes. Surgical care involves many specialties, including general and orthopaedic surgeons, obstetricians and gynecologists, anesthesiologists and numerous other subspecialties. In fact, surgical care does not even always require a surgical specialist. The ability to splint a broken leg, clean a wound, and recognize when to refer an early breast mass can all be accomplished by personnel with limited training, and the effects can be profound. Surgical care also does not need to be expensive to be effective. Most hospitals in LMICs already have an operating room and staff with some training. Basic procedures can often be performed with minimal training, supplies, and equipment.

To best identify and address the deficiencies in global surgical care, a public health approach is useful. To first measure the magnitude of the problem, community surveys of surgical need were conducted in Nepal, Rwanda, and Sierra Leone. With country estimates ranging from 5% to 25%, a conservative estimate is that 350 million people around the world are in need of a surgical consultation and possibly a surgical procedure.

Qualitative studies are also beginning to look at the surgical care knowledge and perception of populations in LMICs. Even people living in the poorest and most remote locations and villages understand the need for surgical care. They want surgical care, but they also know that such care needs to be provided by well-trained and caring practitioners to be done safely.

In an effort to identify the key determinants necessary to implement programs and improve care, hospital-based surveys documenting personnel, infrastructure, procedure, equipment, and supply capacity have been undertaken. The results highlighted the massive deficiencies in the ability to provide safe surgical care. In 2008, Surgeons OverSeas in conjunction with local surgeons and the Sierra Leone Ministry of Health and Sanitation conducted a surgical capacity survey of government hospitals. The results documented, among other things, that only 40% of facilities had the capacity to place a simple drain for chest trauma, and only 30% had running water or eye protection for operating room staff. A comparison with US Civil War hospital data showed that the Sierra Leone facilities were much worse off. Unlike US hospitals in 1864, most facilities in Sierra Leone lacked water, power, advanced anesthesia, and the ability to perform abdominal surgeries and amputations.

Besides the different presentations, varying pathologies, and material deficiencies, there is also the problem of poor access to insufficiently developed health systems in many LMICs. In many communities, if patients are in need of surgical care, if they can get to a health facility, and if there is sufficient infrastructure and personnel, the patient or patient's family receives a written prescription for supplies such as sterile gloves, antibiotics, scalpels, and sutures once a diagnosis is made. The patient or family must then go to an outside pharmacy or market and procure the supplies. If they cannot afford to pay or if the supplies are out of stock, the patient does not receive care. Situations where a woman needing a cesarean section must wait hours or days while her family obtains the money to pay for supplies are not uncommon. The result is frequently the death of the unborn child and possibly the mother; if she survives, she might be left with an ob-stetric fistula. Similar complications also occur with many other potentially treat-able and curable conditions.

To improve surgical care globally and to implement broad and effective proj-ects, clinicians and organizations must first begin with the patient, either with better education in homes and communities or at the patient's bedside. There is an increasing focus on patient-centered care in HICs, and there is no reason why LMICs should be different. Patients should be given a voice to express which sur-gical services are most important to them. Do they want access to only a specific subset of surgical procedures? Should they have access to limited lists of proce-dures determined to be emergency and essential, or should they have access to technologically advanced procedures such as laparoscopic surgery or even trans-plants? As was documented from focus group discussions in Sierra Leone (chap. 1) and described about minimally invasive surgery in Mongolia (chap. 9), patients want the latter.

When discussing surgical care in the developing world, it is the local surgeons, physicians and nurses who are the health-care experts in these settings. They are the ones experienced in providing care in resource-limited environments, deal-ing with their unique cultural concerns and with the ability to understand and confront the political realities. It is the health provider on the ground who must improvise with what they have to treat a surgical condition. They are the ones who must turn away patients because surgical supplies have run out or because a tumor is too advanced to remove safely. They have the best understanding of what the current needs of the local population are, and their concerns must be taken into account if a project is to be successful.

Improving access to surgical care worldwide also requires strong leadership to coordinate efforts. Leaders can come from universities, governments, interna-tional and nongovernmental organizations, or from the general public. Surgical care is still waiting for increased grassroots support, but it is also awaiting a high-profile celebrity advocate. Though frequently controversial, no one can discount the effect that Elton John and Bono have had on raising awareness of HIV or what Princess Diana did for the issue of landmines.

As an increasing number of organizations are incorporating global surgery into their mandate, increased advocacy for surgical care on the public health and global health agendas is urgently required. We must break down the divide between global surgery and global health. Surgical care must be recognized as a valuable adjunct in the treatment of conditions arising from both noncommunicable and communicable diseases. Only through organized efforts and support from the grassroots levels to international institutions will surgical care be recognized as necessary and deemed a political priority.

REFERENCES

Crompton J, Kingham TP, Kamara TB, Brennan MF, Kushner AL. Comparison of surgical care deficiencies between US Civil War hospitals and present-day hospitals in Sierra Leone. *World J Surg.* 2010; 34(8): 1743–47.

Groen RS, Samai M, Stewart KA, et al. Untreated surgical conditions in Sierra Leone: a cluster randomised, cross-sectional, countrywide survey. *Lancet.* 2012; 380(9847): 1082–87.

Groen RS, Sriram VM, Kamara TB, Kushner AL, Blok L. Individual and community perceptions of surgical care in Sierra Leone. *Trop Med Int Health.* 2014; 19(1): 107–16.

Petroze RT, Groen RS, Niyonkuru F, et al. Estimating operative disease prevalence in a low-income country: results of a nationwide population survey in Rwanda. *Surgery.* 2013; 153(4): 457–64.

Page numbers in *italics* refer to figures.